100 Questions & Answers About Gastric Cancer

Manish A. Shah, MD

Division of GI Oncology
Memorial Sloan-Kettering Cancer Center
New York, NY

Natasha Pinheiro, RN

Division of GI Oncology
Memorial Sloan-Kettering Cancer Center
New York, NY

Brinda M. Shah, RPh

New York, NY

JONES AND BARTLETT PUBLISHERS

Sudbury, Massachusetts

BOSTON   TORONTO   LONDON   SINGAPORE

World Headquarters
Jones and Bartlett Publishers
40 Tall Pine Drive
Sudbury, MA 01776
978-443-5000
info@jbpub.com
www.jbpub.com

Jones and Bartlett Publishers
Canada
6339 Ormindale Way
Mississauga, Ontario L5V 1J2
Canada

Jones and Bartlett Publishers
International
Barb House, Barb Mews
London W6 7PA
United Kingdom

Jones and Bartlett's books and products are available through most bookstores and online booksellers. To contact Jones and Bartlett Publishers directly, call 800-832-0034, fax 978-443-8000, or visit our Web site, www.jbpub.com.

Cover Images: *Left Image:* © NorthGeorgiaMedia/ShutterStock, Inc.; *Upper Right Image:* © Diana Lundin/ShutterStock, Inc.; *Middle Right Image:* © Galina Barskaya/ShutterStock, Inc.; *Lower Right Image:* © Yuri Arcurs/ShutterStock, Inc.

Substantial discounts on bulk quantities of Jones and Bartlett's publications are available to corporations, professional associations, and other qualified organizations. For details and specific discount information, contact the special sales department at Jones and Bartlett via the above contact information or send an email to specialsales@jbpub.com.

The authors, editor, and publisher have made every effort to provide accurate information. However, they are not responsible for errors, omissions, or for any outcomes related to the use of the contents of this book and take no responsibility for the use of the products and procedures described. Treatments and side effects described in this book may not be applicable to all people; likewise, some people may require a dose or experience a side effect that is not described herein. Drugs and medical devices are discussed that may have limited availability controlled by the Food and Drug Administration (FDA) for use only in a research study or clinical trial. Research, clinical practice, and government regulations often change the accepted standard in this field. When consideration is being given to use of any drug in the clinical setting, the health care provider or reader is responsible for determining FDA status of the drug, reading the package insert, and reviewing prescribing information for the most up-to-date recommendations on dose, precautions, and contraindications, and determining the appropriate usage for the product. This is especially important in the case of drugs that are new or seldom used.

Production Credits
Executive Publisher: Christopher Davis
Production Director: Amy Rose
Associate Editor: Kathy Richardson
Production Editor: Daniel Stone
Associate Marketing Manager: Rebecca Wasley
Manufacturing Buyer: Therese Connell
Composition: Appingo
Cover Design: Kate Ternullo
Printing and Binding: Malloy, Inc.
Cover Printing: Malloy, Inc.

Library of Congress Cataloging-in-Publication Data
Shah, Manish A.
    100 questions & answers about gastric cancer / Manish A. Shah, Natasha Pinheiro, Brinda M. Shah.
        p. cm.
    ISBN-13: 978-0-7637-5367-2
    ISBN-10: 0-7637-5367-X
    1. Stomach—Cancer—Miscellanea. 2. Stomach—Cancer—Popular works. I. Pinheiro, Natasha. II. Shah, Brinda M. III. Title. IV. Title: One hundred questions and answers about gastric cancer.
    RC280.S8S47 2008
    616.99'433—dc22
                                    2007015591
6048

Printed in the United States of America
11 10 09 08 07   10 9 8 7 6 5 4 3 2 1

I dedicate this handbook to the many patients and families I have encountered and taken care of. Their journey has strengthened my resolve to improve the care of patients with gastric and esophageal cancer. I would like to sincerely thank my parents, Arvind and Sanyukta Shah, for their love and support, without which my career in Medicine would not have flourished. I also dedicate this book to my loving wife, Brinda, and my daughters (Karina, Carisa, and Alyssa) for their affection and understanding.

—**Manish A. Shah, MD**

I would like to dedicate this book to all of the amazing men and women with gastric and gastroesophageal cancers whose care I have been involved with over the last 7 years. They have taught me innumerable life lessons that I will carry with me always. I would also like to give a special thank you to my daughter Chase for being the joy in my life that makes everything else worthwhile.

—**Natasha Pinheiro, RN**

I dedicate this book to my loving husband and three wonderful daughters, Alyssa, Carisa, and Karina. Without their support and understanding, I would not have been able to complete this important project. I would also like to dedicate this book to my parents for their constant love, guidance, and support.

—**Brinda M. Shah, RPh**

Publisher's Note

The authors and publisher would like to gratefully acknowledge the contribution of Jim Vining and Ann Levin, gastric cancer patients who have generously shared their experience, insights, and coping tips, as well as Donna Vining, a cancer patient caregiver. Throughout this book, *Jim's comments*, *Ann's comments*, and *Donna's comments* provide what we hope and expect will be valuable "insider" information for readers from two individuals who have been through the diagnosis, treatment, and recovery from this disease. Thank you Jim, Ann, and Donna.

CONTENTS

This book is dedicated to patients suffering from upper gastrointestinal malignancies, and to their loved ones. Cancers of the gastrointestinal tract make up the majority of all cancers worldwide and are responsible for almost 30% of new cancer diagnoses. Of the GI cancers, stomach, gastroesophageal junction (GEJ), and esophageal cancers are responsible for almost 1/2 of new GI cancer diagnoses. Cancers of the upper gastrointestinal tract (esophagus, GEJ, stomach) are among the most aggressive and difficult to manage malignancies of solid organs. It is our honor to be able to put together, in a concise handbook, answers to the 100 most important and most commonly asked questions about gastric and GEJ cancers.

With this book, we hope to shed some light on the diagnoses and management decisions that physicians make with their patients. As you will see from this handbook—written by a physician, nurse, and pharmacist—the management of upper GI malignancies involves the cooperation of many disciplines. We hope that you will find this book useful, providing resource, information, and support as you meet the challenges inherent in fighting cancer—from its diagnosis to picking a doctor. In addition, while it is impossible to answer all of your questions regarding cancer of the GI tract, it is our hope that you will find the questions/answers provided beneficial in, among other things, dealing with treatment options, the aftermath of a cancer diagnosis, and life with cancer; as well as aiding in the search for support.

We are grateful to Jones and Bartlett for having the insight and recognition of the need for such a book to be offered to people with cancers of the stomach or GEJ.

M.A.S.

N.P.

B.M.S.

PART ONE

The Basics

What is cancer?

What is cancer of the stomach?

What causes cancer of the stomach?

More ...

1. What is cancer?

Cancer is a group of diseases that affect the normal cells of our body. It occurs when a group of normal cells in our body transforms into abnormal cells. These abnormal cells grow and divide out of control until they cause harm to our normal bodily functions.

The **cell** is the building block for all living things. Our body is made up of more than a billion cells. Cells exist in different forms and shapes throughout our body and carry out various specific functions. All of the cells that make up our body come from stem cells. **Stem cells** are special cells that divide into other stem cells and into daughter cells that, with repetitive divisions, may change into different types of cells to carry on different functions. The process of changing from an early stem cell to a more specialized cell that carries on a specific function (like a muscle strand) is called **differentiation**. As cells become more specialized, they become more differentiated. One of the most important characteristics of a normal cell is that it responds to signals from the surrounding environment. Normal cells will grow, divide, and differentiate into more specialized cells in response to growth and differentiation signals. Normal cells will also stop growing and dividing when told to do so, and, importantly, they will also die when they are supposed to. This process of natural death is called **apoptosis**. All cells, except for stem cells, have a specified "life span" and die a natural death of apoptosis when they receive signals to die from surrounding cells. The continuous replacement of old cells for new cells that carry out the same function is a natural and normal aspect of cell growth and division. Another characteristic of normal cells is that they will stop dividing when there are enough normal cells around them to perform their necessary functions. The orderly function of normal cells working together and in harmony a thousand-fold over is the substance of every organ in our body, our bodily systems, and ultimately our body as a whole.

Cancer

An abnormal growth of cells which tends to proliferate in an uncontrolled way. It is a group of diseases that affect the normal cells of our body.

Cell

The smallest unit of living structure capable of independent existence. Cells are highly specialized in structure and function.

Stem cells

Special cells that can turn into any other type of cell in the body.

Differentiation

When describing cancer, refers to how mature a cell appears under the microscope. The more differentiated the cancer cell, the more normal in appearance it is, and the slower it tends to grow. Poorly differentiated or undifferentiated cancer cells lack the structure and function of normal cells.

Apoptosis

Programmed cell death; the natural process by which cells kill themselves.

Cancer occurs when normal cells do not function normally. For example, instead of having a natural life span in which a normal cell dies and allows daughter cells to carry on the function of that cell, a cancer cell no longer responds to signals that tell it to stop functioning and to die. Also, instead of dividing a certain number of times to make a certain number of daughter cells, cancer cells may divide continuously, virtually making an endless supply of daughter cells. Cancer cells therefore live longer and continue to divide and expand. These extra cells form a mass called a **tumor**. Because cancer cells continue to grow and divide, they eventually interfere with the normal functioning of the surrounding noncancerous cells and with the function of that part of the body or organ, inflicting harm on the body as a whole.

Tumors can be benign or malignant. Benign tumors are not cancerous and are rarely life-threatening. Most benign tumors can be removed and do not usually grow back after they are removed. Cells from benign tumors do not spread to other parts of the body or invade the tissues around them. **Malignant tumors** are usually more serious and life-threatening than benign tumors. Malignant tumors can often be removed, but they may return. Cells of malignant tumors can invade and damage nearby organs and tissues.

2. How does a normal cell work, and what causes a normal cell to become cancerous?

The instructions for a normal cell to be normal—that is, to carry out its usual functions—are stored in the genetic material of that cell. This genetic material is called **deoxyribonucleic acid (DNA)** and is passed on from one generation to the next. DNA is stored in every cell in the body. Each cell's DNA carries the instructions for the function of that cell. A cancerous cell develops when these instructions are damaged and altered, making the function of the cell abnormal such that it no longer listens to normal signals that tell it to stop dividing and die.

Cancer occurs when normal cells do not function normally.

Tumor

Any swelling caused by an increased number of abnormal cells.

Benign tumor

A growth or mass of abnormal cells that do not invade or destroy adjacent normal tissue.

Malignant tumor

A growth of abnormal cells that replace normal cells and invade other tissues and organs; growth may recur after attempted removal, and is likely to cause the death of the host if left inadequately treated.

DNA (deoxyribonucleic acid)

A type of nucleic acid found principally in the nuclei of animal and plant cells. It is considered to be the autoreproducing component of chromosomes and many viruses as well as the repository for hereditary characteristics.

The Basics

The stomach is an organ of digestion located just past the esophagus. It lies under the rib cage and diaphragm, and it curls under the liver on the right side of the upper abdomen.

Stomach

An organ of digestion. The stomach begins the digestion process by mixing food with digestive juices, churning it into liquid mulch.

Esophagus

A portion of the digestive canal, shaped like a hollow tube, that connects the throat to the stomach. It is a muscular tube that transfers the bolus of food from the mouth to the stomach. The bolus moves to the stomach independent of gravity—that is, even if you stand on your head, the food you eat will end up in the stomach.

If the cell's DNA gets damaged, the instructions passed on to the cell can also be damaged. DNA can get damaged in many ways, including by environmental toxins, radiation, cigarette smoke, or an inherited mutation in the DNA. As cells divide into daughter cells, they must copy their DNA into two identical sets and then divide such that a copy of each DNA strand is sent to each daughter cell equally. This continual process of replication and division can also lead to DNA damage. Cells routinely identify sections of damaged DNA as they occur and repair them before proceeding with the replication process. It is the balance between DNA damage and repair that tips a normal cell to a cancer cell.

3. How does cancer develop?

Both normal and cancerous cells have a similar structure—there is a nucleus in which the genetic material is stored, and a cytoplasm where the genetic code is translated and the functions of the cell are carried out. As discussed previously, cancer develops when the cell no longer responds to normal signals that tell it to stop functioning, to stop dividing, and to die. Exactly how this can happen is the focus of much worldwide research. The current understanding is that changes or mutations in the genetic code of a cell lead to the changes that make a normal cell cancerous. Thus, if specific sections of DNA are damaged, they can transform a normal cell into a cancer cell.

4. What is the stomach, and what does it do?

The **stomach** is an organ of digestion located just past the esophagus (Figure 1). It lies under the rib cage and diaphragm, and it curls under the liver on the right side of the upper abdomen. Food is passed from the mouth through the **esophagus** and into the stomach. The stomach is where the process of digestion begins. Stomach acids begin to break down the food. The stomach wall, in a series of coordinated contractions, mulches and liquefies the food before it is passed into the intestines, where the nutrients of the food are absorbed.

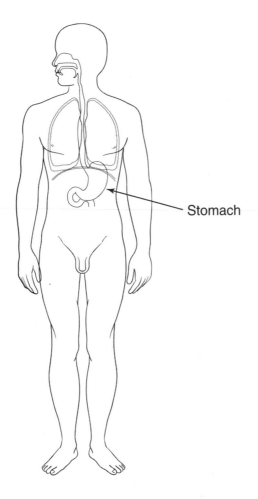

— Stomach

Figure 1   The location of the stomach.

The stomach is a muscular bag that functions primarily as a reservoir, controlling the rate of delivery of the meal to the rest of the gastrointestinal tract. There are three main regions of the stomach: the first portion, the **cardia**, overlaps with the junction between the stomach and esophagus; the second portion, the **fundus**, along with the body forms the bulk of the stomach; and, finally, the **antrum** is the last portion of the stomach (Figure 2). The cardia functions mostly to secrete mucus and bicarbonate, which protects the surface from the corrosive gastric contents. Virtually all of the gastric juices are

Cardia

The first portion of the stomach which overlaps with the junction between the stomach and esophagus.

Fundus

The second portion of the stomach which forms the bulk of the stomach.

Antrum

The last portion of the stomach where food is mixed with gastric juices.

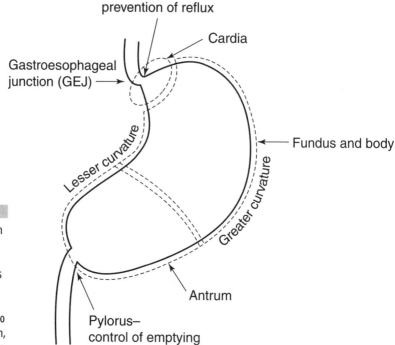

Figure 2   The stomach.

Vitamin B₁₂

An essential vitamin that is important in making red blood cells and DNA; helps with the normal functioning of the nervous system. Also known as cobalamin, deficiency of vitamin B$_{12}$ can result in anemia, peripheral neuropathy with numbness and tingling in the fingertips and toes, loss of appetite, weight loss, and a sore tongue that can sometimes appear smooth and beefy red.

Intrinsic factor

Protein made by the parietal cells of the stomach to help the absorption of vitamin B$_{12}$. Its deficiency is associated with the development of pernicious anemia.

made from specific cells in the fundus. These cells form into small fundic glands that produce the characteristic components of gastric juice—acid and pepsin (a protein substance that digests food). On the other hand, the antrum is where the meal is mixed with the gastric juices and mulched. Eventually, the meal is gradually emptied into the small intestine by a sphincter called the pylorus.

One of the endocrine functions of the stomach is to help absorb **vitamin B$_{12}$**. The parietal cell, which is primarily responsible for the secretion of acid into the gastric juice, is also responsible for secreting **intrinsic factor**. Intrinsic factor is a protein that binds to dietary B$_{12}$ and greatly increases its absorption in the small intestine.

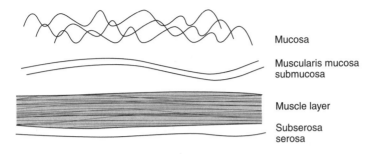

Mucosa

Muscularis mucosa
submucosa

Muscle layer

Subserosa
serosa

Figure 3   Layers of the stomach.

The wall of the stomach is made up of five layers (see Figure 3). The inner layer, the **mucosa**, is where the juices made by the glands help digest food. Most stomach cancers begin in this layer. The **submucosa** is the support tissue for the inner layer. The **muscle layer** creates the motion that is responsible for mixing and mashing food. The **subserosa** is the support tissue for the outer layer. The outer layer, the **serosa**, covers the stomach and holds the stomach in place.

5. What is cancer of the stomach?

Cancer of the stomach occurs when normal cells of the stomach transform into cancerous cells. The term **stomach cancer**, or **gastric cancer**, usually refers to **adenocarcinoma** of the stomach. It is important not to confuse stomach cancer with cancers of the colon, liver, pancreas, or small intestine because they have different symptoms, different outcomes, and different treatments.

Figure 1 identifies the stomach within the chest and abdominal cavity. Cancers of the stomach can occur throughout the lining of the stomach, from the point where the esophagus and stomach meet (the **gastroesophageal junction**, or **GEJ**) all the way to the pylorus where the stomach empties into the duodenum. There are two major types of stomach cancer. The most common type of stomach cancer is called an adenocarcinoma, or gland-forming cancer. This type of stomach cancer

The Basics

Mucosa

The inner layer of the stomach where the juices made by the glands help digest food.

Submucosa

The support tissue for the inner layer of the stomach.

Muscle layer

Creates the motion that is responsible for mixing and mashing food.

Subserosa

The support tissue for the outer layer of the stomach.

Stomach cancer/ gastric cancer

The transformation of normal cells of the stomach into cancerous cells.

Adenocarcinoma

A type of cancer that begins from gland-forming, or secretory, cells.

Gastroesophageal junction (GEJ)

Where the esophagus and stomach meet. It contains the lower esophageal sphincter, which opens and closes, to prevent acid from refluxing into the esophagus.

Gastrointestinal stromal tumor (GIST)

A type of tumor that begins from the cells within the wall of the gastrointestinal tract. Most tumors arise from within the wall of the stomach but can arise anywhere throughout the gastrointestinal tract.

Gastric lymphoma

Cancer of the immune system cells found in the stomach.

Mucosa-associated lymphoid tissue (MALT) lymphoma

A type of cancer that originates from the lymph cells within the lining of the gastrointestinal tract responsible for making antibodies to pathogens. Most MALT lymphomas arise from the stomach and are often caused by infection with *H. pylori*.

Carcinoid tumors

Tumors of hormone-producing cells of the stomach.

Primary cancer

Describes the site of origin of the cancer and generally is described by the organ in which it started.

arises from the functional cells of the stomach and is responsible for about 90% of all stomach cancers. Adenocarcinoma of the stomach is classified in two ways: *intestinal*-type or *diffuse*-type stomach cancer. This is also known as the Lauren's classification. Intestinal gastric cancer tends to grow as tumors within the stomach wall from gland-forming cancer cells. Diffuse stomach cancers grow within the wall as discohesive cells infiltrating throughout.

Another type of stomach cancer is called **gastrointestinal stromal tumor (GIST)** and occurs from the stromal, or supporting, cells of the stomach. GIST tumors are rare tumors that develop from the cells in the wall of the stomach. These cells are called interstitial cells of Cajal. Interstitial cells of Cajal are rare cells that are normally found within the wall of the stomach within the stroma. Their normal function is unknown. GIST tumors can be benign or malignant. These cancers can be found anywhere in the gastrointestinal tract, but they often, in as many as 70% of patients, occur in the stomach.

Other, less common tumors that can be found in the stomach include lymphoma and carcinoid tumors. **Gastric lymphoma** is a cancer of the immune system cells found in the stomach. They usually account for 4% of all stomach cancers. Prognosis and treatment will depend on whether it is an aggressive lymphoma or an indolent, or slow-growing, lymphoma. One type of lymphoma is a **MALT lymphoma**, Mucosa Associated Lymphoid Tissue lymphoma. This lymphoma is caused by immune cells that line the intestines. **Carcinoid tumors** are tumors of hormone-producing cells of the stomach. These tumors generally do not metastasize. Approximately 3% of all stomach cancers are carcinoid tumors.

6. What is the difference between a primary cancer and its metastases?

A **primary cancer** describes the site of origin of the cancer and generally is described by the organ in which it started;

for example, a primary lung cancer is a cancer that started in the lung. As a cancer continues to grow, it may spread into local or regional lymph nodes and then even further to other distant sites. When the cancer does spread to other distant sites, the sites are called **metastases** of the primary tumor. So, for stomach cancer—one that started in the stomach—a common site of spread is the liver. This would then be termed a site of metastasis to the liver. Common sites of spread for stomach cancer include the liver, bone, abdominal cavity, lungs, and brain. If the cancer does spread to these sites, it is still called stomach cancer and is still sensitive to the same treatments used for stomach cancer, even if the cancer is in other organs.

7. What causes stomach cancer?

For the vast majority of patients, stomach cancer is caused by random genetic events, which is "doctor-speak" for bad luck. Essentially, a mutation occurs in the DNA of a stomach cell that lines the inside of the stomach. This mutation is not caught by the cell's repair machinery, and after many replications and more mutations, eventually the first cancer cell develops, which then leads to the cancer itself. This cancer cell carries with it the basic properties of cancer—that of continuously growing and producing more cancer cells and avoiding programmed cell death, which was discussed earlier.

There are associations linked to the development of stomach cancer as well. For example, about 10% to 15% of all stomach cancers are inherited. There is also an association between stomach cancer and a bacterial infection of the stomach called **Helicobacter pylori.** *H. Pylori* infection causes inflammation, and the stomach cells are damaged by cells of the immune system. It is not known exactly why this condition progresses to cancer, but it may be related to the irritation caused by chronic inflammation.

Obesity, chronic heartburn, and tobacco and alcohol use are other characteristics associated with the development of

The Basics

Metastasis

A term that describes the spread of cancer from one part of the body to another. A tumor formed by cells that have spread is called a metastatic tumor or a metastasis. The tumor cells at a metastatic site contain cells that are like those of the primary cancer.

Helicobacter pylori (H. pylori)

A bacteria that causes inflammation and irritation of the lining of the stomach and intestine. Infection with *H. pylori* can cause ulceration of the stomach and different types of stomach cancer, including gastric adenocarcinoma and MALT lymphoma.

stomach cancer. It is important to realize that not all patients with these characteristics will indeed develop the disease. Eating fruits and vegetables reduces the risk of developing stomach cancer.

A stomach ulcer is not, by itself, associated with a high risk of stomach cancer. However, it may be an indicator that other risk factors for stomach cancer exist, such as infection with *H. pylori* or reflux disease, as these are also risk factors for stomach ulcers. Please understand that the majority of patients with gastric ulcers do not go on to develop stomach cancer.

8. How fast does stomach cancer develop?

It is thought that over many years the lining of the stomach may change gradually due to chronic irritation. These changes in the lining are called precancerous changes.

It is not entirely clear how fast stomach cancer develops. It is thought that over many years the lining of the stomach may change gradually due to chronic irritation. These changes in the lining are called *precancerous changes*.

Superficial gastritis occurs from inflammation of the stomach lining. In this phase, the stomach lining is often trying to repair itself, and there is a large amount of regeneration seen under the microscope. This can lead to *atrophic gastritis*, whereby the gland-forming cells of the stomach lining (that is, those that produce acid) burn out and are no longer found, or are absent, within the stomach wall. The next sequential step is *metaplasia*. This is a precancerous change in which the normal lining of the stomach is replaced with cells that resemble those that line the intestine. Finally, *dysplasia* can develop with continued, chronic irritation. In this phase, cells appear even more abnormal, particularly with regard to size, shape, and orientation within the stomach wall. Dysplasia is felt to be a precursor lesion to stomach cancer.

It may take years for the lining of the stomach to change from superficial gastritis to dysplasia. However, once stomach cancer begins, it is felt to be an aggressive cancer that can grow relatively rapidly over the course of 1 to 2 years.

9. How common is stomach cancer?

Stomach cancer is one of the most common diseases world-wide. About 975,000 new cases of stomach cancer were diagnosed worldwide in the year 2000. It is the third most prevalent disease worldwide, and it was responsible for about 734,000 deaths in the year 2000. In the United States, there will be about 21,260 new cases of stomach cancer diagnosed in 2007, and about 11,210 people (6610 men and 4600 women) will die of this disease. Two thirds of those who have stomach cancer are 65 years or older. The risk of a person getting stomach cancer in his or her lifetime is about 1 in 100.

Stomach cancer is more common worldwide, particularly in less-developed countries. It is the second-leading cause of cancer-related deaths in the world. Stomach cancer used to be a leading cause of cancer deaths in the United States, but now it is much less common. The reasons for this decrease in the incidence of stomach cancer are not completely known, but they may be linked to increased use of refrigeration for food storage and decreased use of salted and smoked foods. Some doctors believe the major reason that stomach cancer has decreased is because of the frequent use of antibiotics to treat infections in children. In addition to treating the intended infection, antibiotics could have killed *H. pylori* bacteria, which is a major cause of stomach cancer.

Stomach cancer used to be a leading cause of cancer deaths in the United States, but now it is much less common.

10. Is there a difference in epidemiology between stomach and gastroesophageal junction cancer?

The incidence of cancer of the gastroesophageal junction (GEJ) is rising at an alarming rate in the United States. This is a cancer of the area between the stomach and the esophagus. Cancers of the cardia of the stomach and of the lower esophagus are often grouped together with the GEJ. Over the last 30 years, we have noticed a shift in the epidemiology of stomach and GEJ cancers. Specifically, while the incidence of stomach cancers has decreased over the past 30 years, in that same time span, cancers of the GEJ have risen significantly. Although the incidence remains almost twice as high in African Americans and Hispanics as compared to Caucasians, the rise has been much more prominent in white Americans, particularly young, white, affluent males. Also, the risk of stomach cancer is about two-fold higher in males than females, but for cancers of the GEJ, the risk of developing cancer is four- to five-fold higher in males than in females. The reason for the difference between stomach and GEJ adenocarcinomas is unknown and is the subject of much research.

11. How does stomach cancer spread?

Stomach cancer begins on the inside wall of the stomach. It then spreads through the wall and often into lymph nodes next to the stomach. Cancer of the stomach can then spread directly to the *peritoneal cavity*, which is the abdominal space that holds the intestines (Figure 4). The peritoneal cavity is covered by a soft tissue blanket called the *omentum*. Stomach cancer often spreads directly from the stomach and regional lymph nodes to the omentum. This type of spread is by direct extension.

Cancer of the stomach can also spread via the blood system (circulation) to other sites in the body. The most common site of spread by circulation is to the liver. Other common sites of spread include the lungs, bone, and brain. Cancer of the stomach can also spread by lymphatics to other lymph nodes that are more distant from the stomach than the regional lymph nodes (Figure 4).

When stomach cancer spreads by direct extension to the peritoneum or to distant lymph nodes, or via blood circulation to other organs within the body, it is still termed stomach cancer, but it is cancer that has metastasized. For example, if stomach cancer spreads to the liver, it is still called and treated as metastatic stomach cancer, and it may be referred to as a "distant" tumor.

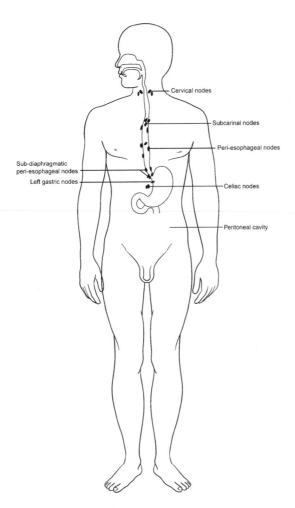

Figure 4   Lymph nodes and peritoneum.

12. What are lymph nodes?

Lymph is the semiclear fluid in the body that drains waste from normal cells. This fluid travels throughout the body by lymph vessels to lymph nodes. **Lymph nodes**, or lymph glands, are small, beanlike structures that are located through-out the body. Lymph nodes filter unwanted substances, such as bacteria and cancer cells, from this fluid. Within lymph nodes are cells of the immune system, including white blood

Lymph nodes

Small, beanlike structures located throughout the body that filter unwanted substances such as bacteria from lymph.

13

cells such as T-cells and B-cells. It is important to check lymph nodes during diagnosis and treatment because they filter cancer cells (Figure 5).

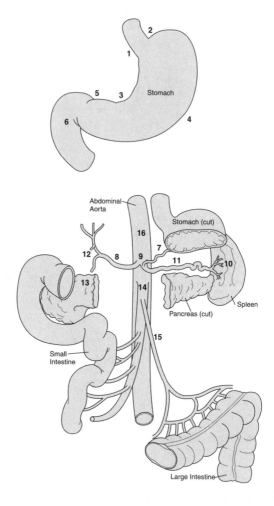

Figure 5   Japanese Research Society Nodal Classification. Classification and anatomic location of lymph node groups. Involvement of nodes along the lesser or greater curvature (groups 1–6) constitutes N1 disease, and the celiac axis and its three branches are N2 (7–11), N3 (12–14), and N4 (15, 16). N1: 1, right paracardial; 2, left paracardial; 3, lesser curvature; 4, greater curvature; 5, suprapyloric; 6, infrapyloric. N2: 7, left gastric artery; 8, common hepatic artery; 9, celiac artery; 10, splenic hilus; 11, splenic artery. N3: 12, hepatic pedicle; 13, retropancreatic; 14, mesenteric root. N4: 15, middle colic artery; 16, para-aortic. .

PART TWO

Risk and Prevention

Can I prevent stomach cancer?

What are the risk factors for stomach cancer?

What are the warning signs for stomach cancer?

More . . .

13. Can I prevent stomach cancer?

We don't know yet how to prevent stomach cancer. Avoiding risk factors when possible may lower your risk, but this cannot guarantee protection from the disease.

We don't know yet how to prevent stomach cancer. Avoiding risk factors when possible may lower your risk, but this cannot guarantee protection from the disease. Early detection is the best way to improve your chance of successful treatment. You can reduce your risk by reducing your alcohol intake and by not smoking. You should avoid a diet high in smoked or pickled foods, salted meats, or foods preserved in nitrates. Eating a diet rich in fruits and vegetables may reduce the risk of getting stomach cancer. The American Cancer Society recommends eating a variety of healthy foods with an emphasis on plant sources.

14. What are risk factors?

Risk factor

Anything that increases a person's risk of getting a disease.

Anything that increases your risk of getting a disease is called a **risk factor**. Having risk factors for a particular disease does not mean that you will definitely get the disease. Some risk factors are environmental, while others may be genetic. We may have some control over our environmental factors (smoking, chemical exposure, pollution) and may be able to minimize our exposure, and therefore our risk. Genetic factors are those that we inherit and have no control over. Often, the cause of a disease is not simply one risk factor, but the combination of multiple factors that you may or may not be aware of.

15. What are the risk factors for stomach cancer?

There are many known risk factors for stomach cancer. How these factors cause cells of the stomach lining to become cancerous is the subject of ongoing research.

Helicobacter pylori infection: The *H. pylori* bacterium infects millions of people worldwide and is a major cause of stomach cancer. Long-term infection of the stomach with *H. pylori* may lead to chronic inflammation and damage to the inner layer of the stomach. This chronic inflammation may result in precancerous changes to the lining of the stomach. Patients with adenocarcinoma of the stomach have a higher rate of infection than those without cancer. Some strains of *H. pylori* are more commonly associated with the development of stomach cancer than other strains. *H. pylori* infection is also associated with some types of lymphoma of the stomach (for example, MALT lymphoma). The exact mechanism by which infection with *H. pylori* leads to the development of stomach cancer is not well understood. Indeed, the vast majority of people who are infected with *H. pylori* never develop cancer of the stomach.

Dietary causes: People whose diets contain large amounts of smoked foods, salted fish and meat, and pickled vegetables have an increased risk of getting stomach cancer. Nitrates and nitrites are substances commonly found in cured meats, some drinking water, and certain vegetables. These nitrates and nitrites can be converted by *H. pylori* into compounds that have been found to cause stomach cancer in animals. Eating whole-grain products and fresh fruits and vegetables rich in vitamins A and C appears to lower the risk of stomach cancer.

Tobacco and alcohol abuse: Smoking increases stomach cancer risk, particularly for cancers of the proximal stomach (the upper portion of the stomach closest to the esophagus). The rate of stomach cancer is approximately doubled in smokers. Some studies have linked alcohol use to stomach cancer, but this is not certain.

Obesity: Obesity is a major cause of many cancers and especially cancers of the cardia (part nearest the esophagus) of the stomach. Obesity is related to increased reflux and irritation of the lining of the stomach, particularly in the cardia or lower esophagus.

Previous stomach surgery: Stomach cancers are more likely to develop in those who have had part of their stomach removed to treat noncancerous conditions such as ulcers. This may be due to the presence of more nitrite-producing bacteria. Acid production goes down after ulcer surgery, and there may be reflux (backup) of bile from the small intestine into the stomach. The risk continues to increase for as long as 15 to 20 years following surgery and for those patients who underwent a Billroth II operation, in which the pyloris of the stomach is removed. This operation reduces the acid production of the stomach.

Pernicious anemia

The result of a vitamin B_{12} deficiency.

Pernicious anemia: **Pernicious anemia** occurs as a result of a vitamin B_{12} deficiency. There are certain cells in the lining of the stomach that normally produce a protein necessary for absorbing vitamin B_{12} from foods. If enough of this substance, called **intrinsic factor**, is not present, a vitamin B_{12} deficiency results, leading to anemia (a problem in producing enough red blood cells). In addition to anemia, there is an increased risk of stomach cancer for patients with this disease. Because the risk for developing stomach cancer from a vitamin B_{12} deficiency seems to be very small, screening these patients for stomach cancer is not recommended.

Intrinsic factor

Protein made by the parietal cells of the stomach to help the absorption of vitamin B_{12}. Its deficiency is associated with the development of pernicious anemia.

Menetrier disease

Hyperproliferative disorders of the stomach caused by dysregulated receptor tyrosine kinases (RTKs).

Menetrier disease: Also known as hypertrophic gastropathy, **Menetrier disease** is a condition of the large folds in the stomach. It is associated with changes in the stomach lining and low acid production. Because this disease is very rare, the exact risk of stomach cancer is not known.

Gender: Stomach cancer is more than twice as common in men as it is in women.

Most people diagnosed with stomach cancer are in their late 60s, 70s, and 80s.

Ethnicity: Stomach cancer is more common in Hispanics and African Americans than in non-Hispanic whites. It is most common in Asian/Pacific Islanders.

Aging: There is a sharp increase in stomach cancer after the age of 50. Most people diagnosed with stomach cancer are in their late 60s, 70s, and 80s.

Type A blood: Blood type groups refer to certain antigens that are normally present on red blood cells and some other types of cells. Antigens are chemicals that are recognized by the immune system. These groups are important in matching blood for transfusions. For reasons unknown, people with type A blood have a higher risk of developing stomach cancer.

Familial cancer syndromes: **Hereditary nonpolyposis colorectal cancer** (also known as HNPCC or Lynch syndrome) and **familial adenomatous polyposis** (also known as FAP) are inherited genetic disorders. People affected with these inherited genetic disorders and mutations have a greatly increased risk of developing colorectal cancer and a slightly increased risk of developing stomach cancer. People who carry mutations of the inherited breast cancer genes *BRCA1* and *BRCA2* may also have a higher rate of stomach cancer. Recently, **Diffuse Hereditary Gastric Cancer** has been discovered as a new familial cancer syndrome for the development of diffuse stomach cancer. In this syndrome, patients from the same family who develop stomach cancer develop the diffuse type of stomach cancer, more often at an early age (younger than 50 years). The gene responsible for diffuse hereditary stomach cancer is *CDH1*, which is the gene for a cell surface protein called E-cadherin.

Family history of stomach cancer: People with several first-degree relatives who have had stomach cancer are more likely to develop this disease.

Stomach polyps: **Polyps** are growths on the lining of the stomach that can turn into cancer. Most types of polyps (such as hyperplastic polyps or inflammatory polyps) do not appear to increase a person's risk of stomach cancer. Adenomatous-type polyps (adenomas) can sometimes develop into cancer.

Geography: Stomach cancer is most common in Japan, China, Southern and Eastern Europe, and South and Central America. This disease is least common in Northern and Western

Risk and Prevention

Hereditary nonpolyposis colorectal cancer

A hereditary syndrome that significantly increases the risk of many cancers including the colon and stomach. Unlike FAP, it is not characterized by numerous polyps.

Familial adenomatous polyposis (FAP)

A hereditary syndrome that significantly increases the risk of colon cancer and also stomach cancer. It is characterized by thousands of polyps in the intestines.

Diffuse Hereditary Gastric Cancer

A hereditary syndrome in which affected individuals have an increased risk of developing diffuse gastric cancer.

Polyps

A growth in the lining of the intestines. They come in a variety of shapes and carry a varying risk of developing into a cancer.

19

Africa, South Central Asia, and North America. The cause for this geographic variation is not clear. The incidence of diffuse stomach cancer (Lauren's classification) is constant across the globe, at a rate of about 1 to 2 per 100,000 people. Unlike diffuse stomach cancer, the rate of intestinal-type stomach cancer varies across the globe and is most prevalent in areas with the highest rates of stomach cancer. For example, in Japan, where the prevalence of stomach cancer is one of the highest worldwide, the rate of intestinal stomach cancer is also among the highest in the world, whereas the rate of diffuse stomach cancer in Japan is the same as everywhere else in the world.

Epstein-Barr virus: This virus causes infectious mononucleosis. Almost all adults have been infected with this virus at some time in their lives, usually as children or adolescents. It has been linked to some forms of lymphoma. Epstein-Barr virus has also been found in the stomach cancers of about 5% to 10% of people with this disease. These people tend to have a slower-growing, less aggressive cancer with a lower tendency to spread. It is unclear what role the virus plays in the development of stomach cancer.

16. Is stomach cancer hereditary?

Most stomach cancers are not hereditary. It is estimated that 85% of stomach cancer worldwide comes from "**sporadic**" **mutations**, that is, mutations that do not run in families. Conversely, about 15% of stomach cancers *do* occur in families with a family history of the disease. Recently, a syndrome of hereditable stomach cancer called Diffuse Hereditary Stomach Cancer was discovered (see Question 15). In this disease, all family members who get the disease develop the diffuse type of stomach cancer, often at a young age (younger than age 50). This syndrome is responsible for about 5% of all hereditable stomach cancers. The other familial cancer syndromes that can lead to stomach cancer include hereditary

Most stomach cancers are not hereditary. It is estimated that 85% of stomach cancer worldwide comes from sporadic mutations, that is, mutations that do not run in families.

Sporadic mutation

A genetic mutation that occurs the first time in a family or a new mutation that is not likely to occur again within a family.

nonpolyposis colorectal cancer (also known as HNPCC or Lynch syndrome) and familial adenomatous polyposis (also known as FAP) (see Question 15). For patients with FAP, the risk of stomach cancer is ten-fold higher than the general population. Both of these syndromes are rare.

The remaining approximately 10% of hereditable stomach cancer syndromes are of unknown genetic cause. This is an area of active research.

17. What are the warning signs for stomach cancer?

Most cases of early stomach cancer do not present with clear symptoms. As the cancer grows and spreads, the most common symptoms are discomfort in the stomach area, feeling full or bloated after a small meal, blood in the stool, unexplained weight loss, loss of appetite, heartburn or indigestion, and nausea and vomiting. Most patients have symptoms for 3 to 9 months before being diagnosed with the disease.

In more advanced cases of stomach cancer, symptoms may include **jaundice** (yellowing of the eyes and skin), **ascites** (fluid buildup in the abdominal area), and having trouble swallowing. Some of these symptoms can occur with noncancerous conditions, such as a stomach virus, or with other types of cancer. Often these symptoms are not due to cancer, but it is always best to check with your health care provider.

18. Are there any screening guidelines for the early detection of stomach cancer?

A successful screening program requires that the disease is prevalent in the population. Because stomach cancer has declined in the United States and most Western countries, there are no effective screening guidelines in the West. However, in areas where stomach cancer is more prevalent (such as Japan),

The most common symptoms of stomach cancer are discomfort in the stomach area, feeling full or bloated after a small meal, blood in the stool, unexplained weight loss, loss of appetite, heartburn or indigestion, and nausea and vomiting.

Jaundice

Yellowish discoloration of the skin and eyes caused by accumulation of bilirubin.

Ascites

An abnormal accumulation of fluid in the abdomen.

Risk and Prevention

21

Upper endoscopy

Examination of the inside of the stomach using an endoscope; a thin, tube-like instrument with a light and a lens for viewing; passed through the mouth and esophagus.

active screening for the disease is advocated. Screening is usually performed by an **upper endoscopy** so that the lining of the stomach can be examined under direct inspection.

Some recent research has examined the usefulness of screening other high-risk populations besides Japan. Identifying a population at high risk may allow endoscopy screening to be more cost effective and may identify stomach cancer at an earlier stage when chances for curing the disease are higher.

PART THREE

Diagnosis and Staging

What tests are performed to aid in the diagnosis of cancer?

What is stomach cancer staging?

I've just been diagnosed with stomach cancer. What is the usual way to stage my disease?

More . . .

19. What tests are performed to aid in the diagnosis of cancer?

A complete medical history is the first step in determining your general health. In such an interview, your doctor will ask you questions about your risk factors, symptoms, and lifestyle that might suggest a diagnosis of stomach cancer. He or she may also ask you questions about your general health in case you need to have surgery.

A physical exam will also provide the doctor with your general health status, signs of stomach cancer, and other health problems. Important parts of a physical examination include examining the heart, lungs, and abdomen. Other areas examined include your lymph nodes, your throat, your nervous system function, and your arms and legs for pulses and swelling. The medical history and physical examination are critical parts of a doctor's evaluation and may provide clues to the diagnosis of your disease. It will also determine your general health and assess your suitability for surgery or chemotherapy.

The most common procedure or test used to diagnose stomach cancer is an endoscopy.

The most common procedure or test used to diagnose stomach cancer is an endoscopy (see Question 20). An upper endoscopy is performed while you are asleep. Biopsies or tissue samples may also be taken by a small instrument through the endoscope. The tissue sample is examined under a microscope to determine whether cancer is present. This biopsy will also help to determine what type of cancer is present.

Stomach cancer can appear as an ulcer, a mushroom-shaped mass, or a flat, thickened area of mucosa known as *linitis plastica*. This is more difficult to recognize in early stages, and only a biopsy of this area will produce an accurate diagnosis.

Imaging studies such as barium contrast enhanced upper gastrointestinal radiographs, endoscopic ultrasounds, computed tomography, positron emission tomography, magnetic resonance imaging, and chest x-rays may be performed, as discussed next.

- A *barium contrast enhanced upper gastrointestinal radiograph* is a test in which you drink a barium-containing solution that coats the lining of your esophagus, stomach, and first part of the small intestine (called an upper GI series). The radiologist will take x-ray pictures that show an outline of the lining of these organs. Any irregular surfaces or strictures may lead to further studies to identify the abnormality. To determine early stomach cancer, a "double contrast" technique is used.
- *Ultrasonography* uses sound waves to produce images of organs. A transducer emits sound waves and detects the echoes from the internal organs. This pattern of echoes is processed by a computer to create an image. An endoscopic ultrasound is done by placing a probe into the stomach through the mouth or nose. It is used to estimate how far the cancer has spread into the wall of the stomach, to other tissues, or to the lymph nodes.
- *Computed tomography (CT)* or *computed assisted tomography (CAT)* is an x-ray that shows detailed cross-sectional images of your body. A machine called a CT scanner rotates around you, taking many pictures of multiple slices of the part of the body being studied, and then the computer combines these pictures to make an image. The CT scans show the stomach fairly clearly and can usually confirm the location of the cancer. It can also show areas near the stomach where the cancer may have spread. The CT scan can help determine whether surgery would be a good option. CT scans can also be used to guide a biopsy needle to help detect metastasis.
- *Positron emission tomography (PET)* is a test in which radioactive glucose is injected into the vein. Because cancer cells use up sugar faster than normal tissue cells, the cancerous tissue takes up the radioactive material. A scanner then spots the radioactive deposits. This is

useful in determining cancer that has spread beyond the stomach and can't be removed by surgery. It is also useful for cancer staging. Although the majority of stomach cancers will take up the radioactive sugar and be visible on a PET scan, about one-third of stomach cancers do not, and thus are considered not-avid. The radioactive sugar is called FDG, 18-fluorodeoxyglucose, and stomach cancers that do not take up this radio-activity are called non-FDG avid. Diffuse stomach cancers, or stomach cancers that start farther away from the esophagus, are more likely not to be FDG-avid. If the PET scan does not show any abnormal uptake, it may mean that the cancer is no longer visible (if it once was visible on a PET scan before), or simply that the type of cancer you have does not take up FDG, in which case the scan is considered to be noninformative.

- *Magnetic resonance imaging (MRI)* uses radio waves and strong magnets. The energy from these waves is absorbed and released in a pattern that is consistent with certain tissues and diseases. A computer translates the patterns of waves into a detailed image slice that is parallel with the length of the body.

- *Chest x-rays* can also determine whether the cancer has spread to the lungs or whether there are any serious lung or heart diseases present. In modern practice, a CT scan of the chest is more often performed to identify disease in the lungs.

Laparoscopy

Examination of the interior of the abdomen by means of a laparoscope.

Peritoneum

The tissue that lines the abdominal wall and most of the structures and organs within the abdomen.

A **laparoscopy** may be performed in preparation for surgery by a surgeon. The laparoscope is a thin, flexible tube that is inserted through a small surgical opening, and it transmits a picture of the inside of the abdomen to a monitor. This can help identify the spread of cancer to the surface of the intestines, called the **peritoneum**. Often, radiographic imaging studies, including CT scan, PET scan, and MRIs, are unable to identify disease that has spread to the peritoneum. In the United States, about one-third of stomach cancers that are felt to be localized to the stomach and lymph nodes next to the stomach have in fact spread to the surface of the bowel, and they are identified only by laparoscopy.

Laboratory tests, including a complete blood count (CBC) to look for anemia and a fecal occult blood test to detect blood in stool, may also be performed. Tests that measure the levels of CA19-9 or CEA in the blood may indicate the presence of cancer. These substances are released into the bloodstream from both cancer cells and normal cells. When the levels of these substances are higher than normal amounts, this can be a sign of stomach cancer or other conditions. There will also be routine tests to determine liver function. The doctor may recommend other tests and procedures too.

20. What is an EGD, and how is it done?

Stomach cancer is most commonly diagnosed by an upper endoscopy. This test is also known as an **esophagogastroduodenoscopy**, or **EGD**. An EGD is an examination of the lining of the esophagus, stomach, and upper duodenum with a small camera (flexible endoscope) that is inserted down the throat.

Esophagogastro-duodenoscopy

An examination of the lining of the esophagus, stomach, and upper duodenum with a flexible tube that has a small camera on the end and that is inserted down the throat.

Before the test begins, you will be given a sedative and a pain medication. A local anesthetic will be sprayed into your mouth to suppress the need to cough or gag while the endoscope is inserted. A mouth guard will be inserted to protect your teeth and the endoscope. If you wear dentures, they will need to be removed before starting the procedure.

In most cases, an intravenous line will be inserted into your arm to administer medications during the procedure. You will be instructed to lie on your left side.

After the gag reflex has been suppressed by the anesthetic, the endoscope will be advanced through the esophagus to the stomach and duodenum. Air will be introduced through the endoscope to enhance viewing. The lining of the esophagus, stomach, and upper duodenum are examined, and biopsies are obtained through the endoscope. Biopsies are tissue samples that are reviewed under the microscope.

After the test is completed, food and liquids will be restricted until your gag reflex returns. The test lasts about 5 to 20 minutes. To prepare for the test, you will be required to fast overnight (6 to 12 hours before the test). You will also sign an informed consent. You may be told to stop aspirin and other blood-thinning medications for several days before the test.

Jim's comment:

Be sure to take someone with you so that he or she can drive you home, or be prepared to stay at the hospital for several hours while the anesthetic wears off. I have heard that people are scared of this procedure, and there is really no reason to be scared. You never feel anything, and the biopsies (both cancerous and healthy) are very important tissues that are greatly needed to make the correct diagnosis and possibly also in the research departments.

21. What is meant by cancer staging?

Cancer staging is a medical term referring to the extent of cancer in your body and how far the cancer has spread. Doctors use staging as a way to communicate to others the status of a cancer. The staging system includes where it is located, the extent of the disease, and whether it has spread to any lymph nodes or other organ systems in the body. Generally, patients with early stage cancers have the disease localized to the site where the tumor originated. With more advanced stages, the tumor is more extensive, eventually reaching stage IV, which is metastatic. Treatment options are determined based on the stage of your cancer.

22. What is stomach cancer staging?

The extent of spread of stomach cancer is the most important factor in selecting treatment options and estimating the

Generally, patients with early stage cancers have the disease localized to the site where the tumor originated. With more advanced stages, the tumor is more extensive, eventually reaching stage IV, which is metastatic. Treatment options are determined based on the stage of your cancer.

Cancer staging

The process to identify the extent of cancer in the body. The stage is usually determined by the depth of penetration into the wall, the involvement of lymph nodes next to the cancer, and whether the cancer has traveled from the primary origin to metastatic sites of disease.

course of a patient's illness and outlook for recovery and survival (prognosis). The stage of a cancer can be determined by the information gathered before surgery (clinical stage) or from the results of the surgery and the pathologist's assessment of the removed tissues (pathologic stage). The stages described below are the pathologic stages, determined by the results of surgery.

The system most often used to stage stomach cancer in the United States is the American Joint Commission on Cancer (AJCC) TNM system. T stands for features of the tumor (how far it has grown within the stomach and into nearby organs), N stands for spread to lymph nodes, and M is for metastasis (spread) to distant organs. In TNM staging, information about the tumor, lymph nodes, and metastasis is combined in a process called *stage grouping*.

Table 1   Staging for stomach cancer (AJCC 2002)

Stage	T	N	M
0	in situ	0	0
Ia	1	0	0
Ib	2 1	0 1	0 0
II	2 1 3	1 2 0	0 0 0
IIIa	2 3 4	2 1 0	0 0 0
IIIb	3	2	0
IV	4 Any Any	1–2 3 Any	0 0 1

N1 = 1 to 6 lymph nodes involved, N2 = 7 to 15 lymph nodes involved, and N3 = more than 15 lymph nodes involved.

After the T, N, and M stages of a stomach cancer have been determined, this information is combined and expressed as a stage, ranging from stage I through IV in the AJCC system.

Stage 0

This is cancer in its earliest stage. It has not grown beyond the layer of cells that line the stomach (epithelium). This stage is also known as carcinoma in situ, which means the cancer cells are in the innermost layer, where they started.

Stage IA

The cancer has grown under the epithelium into the next layer, the lamina propria or the submucosa. However, it has not grown into the main muscle layer of the stomach, called the muscularis. The cancer has not spread to any lymph nodes or anywhere else.

Stage IB

Two combinations of T and N features are assigned to this stage:

1. Just as in stage IA, the cancer has grown under the epithelium into submucosa, but it has not grown into the muscularis, the main muscle layer of the stomach. It has spread to as many as six lymph nodes near the stomach, but not to any other tissues or organs, or
2. The cancer has grown into the main muscle layer of the stomach wall, called the muscularis, and may have grown into the subserosa (outermost layer of the stomach wall). It has not spread to any other tissues or organs and has not spread to any lymph nodes.

Stage II

Three combinations of T and N features are assigned to this stage.

1. The cancer has grown under the epithelium into the submucosa. It has not grown into the muscular layer, but it has spread to between 7 and 15 lymph nodes near the stomach, or
2. The cancer has grown into the muscular layer and may have grown into the subserosa (outermost layer of the stomach wall). It has not spread to any nearby tissues or organs, but it has spread to between 1 and 6 lymph nodes near the stomach, or
3. The cancer has grown through all the layers to the outside of the stomach. It has not spread to any nearby tissues or organs and has not spread to any lymph nodes.

Stage IIIA

Three combinations of T and N features are assigned to this stage:

1. The cancer has grown into the muscular layer and may have spread into the subserosa. It has not spread to any nearby tissues or organs, but it has spread to between 7 and 15 lymph nodes near the stomach, or
2. The cancer has grown completely through the muscular layer and the subserosa to the outside of the stomach. It has not spread to any nearby tissues or organs, but it has spread to between 1 and 6 lymph nodes near the stomach, or
3. The cancer has grown completely through the stomach wall into other nearby organs, such as the spleen, liver, intestines, kidneys, or pancreas. It has not spread to any lymph nodes.

Stage IIIB

The cancer has grown completely through the muscular layer and the subserosa. It has not spread to any nearby tissues or organs, but it has spread to between 7 and 15 lymph nodes near the stomach.

Stage IV

1. The cancer has grown completely through the stomach wall directly into other nearby organs, such as the spleen, liver, intestines, kidneys, or pancreas, and spread to any lymph node.
2. The cancer has spread to more than 15 lymph nodes, or
3. The cancer has spread to other organs such as the liver, lungs, brain, or bones.

23. I've just been diagnosed with stomach cancer. What is the usual way to stage my disease?

You've had an endoscopy to establish that you have cancer of the stomach. After a medical history and physical examination, your physician will often perform basic laboratory tests, which include a complete blood count and assessment of your kidney and liver functions. The next step, usually, is a CT scan of the chest, abdomen, and pelvis. If there are abnormalities in organs other than the stomach, these will need to be better evaluated. This means that you may undergo additional testing such as an MRI or PET scan. Also, generally a biopsy is performed by a needle under CT scan guidance to confirm that a site outside the stomach has stomach cancer. If no other sites are identified, then you may have localized stomach cancer. Often, however, stomach cancer can spread to the **peritoneum**, the surface of the intestines, and it is often not well visualized on imaging studies such as CT, MRI, or PET scans. In this case, to make sure the cancer hasn't spread to the peritoneum, a laparoscopy is performed. At the conclusion of these tests, you should know the extent of your cancer and

Peritoneum

The tissue that lines the abdominal wall and most of the structures and organs within the abdomen.

where it may have spread. The next step is finding the right therapy.

24. Is it possible I have a different type of cancer?

One of the most important things to do is to make sure your pathology report is reviewed and confirmed by experts in gastrointestinal pathology. There are many different types of stomach cancer (see Question 5). It is important to understand that the specific type of stomach cancer diagnosed may alter the treatment plan. Also, on rare occasions, a cancer in the lining of the stomach may not have originated in the stomach; that is, the stomach may not be the primary site of the tumor. For example, breast cancer has been known to spread to the stomach. Reviewing the pathology of the endoscopic biopsy and comparing it with a previous malignancy may aid in confirming whether the cancer in the stomach is the primary site of malignancy or a site of metastases. It is important to do this because different types of cancers have different treatments.

There are many different types of stomach cancer. It is important to understand that the specific type of stomach cancer diagnosed may alter the treatment plan.

PART FOUR

Coping with the Diagnosis

I've been diagnosed with stomach cancer, what do I do now?

Should I get a second opinion?

How do I emotionally handle a new cancer diagnosis?

More . . .

25. I've been diagnosed with stomach cancer. What do I do now?

If you were diagnosed by an internist or gastroenterologist, the first thing you need to do is find a cancer specialist. If you do not have a referral from your doctor, you may need to find a specialist on your own (see Question 26). Generally, if your cancer has spread to metastatic sites, you will want to see a medical oncologist first. However, if your cancer seems localized, you may see either a medical oncologist or a surgical oncologist first. Other important things to do and/or be aware of include:

- Learn about stomach cancer so that you will be able to make well-informed decisions. You may use the Internet (see Questions 26 and 83) to learn about stomach cancer and its treatment.
- Know your pertinent health and medication history prior to going to see a cancer specialist.
- Call your insurance company to find out what benefits you have regarding specialized cancer care. You should also know whether you need to obtain any prior authorization for seeing a specialist and for obtaining any tests that may be performed.
- Have a support system of family or friends to go with you to your doctors' appointments. Designate a family member or friend to help you navigate any insurance issues that may arise.
- Find a support group for patients with stomach cancer so that you can talk to other people about their experiences with the disease and/or treatment.

26. How do I choose a doctor, oncologist, or surgeon?

When you have been given a possible gastric cancer diagnosis, it is essential to initiate care with an appropriately trained physician or specialist. There are a number of steps that aid in this process.

1. You can speak with your primary care physician to get referrals for cancer care specialists. A recommendation from a reliable source, such as your gastroenterologist, would also be a good place to start.
2. You should confirm with your insurance carrier whether there are any restrictions to specialized care.
3. Investigate online cancer care Web sites (American Cancer Society, Cancer Care, and National Cancer Institute) and hospital Web sites to get a list of physicians that specialize in gastric cancer (see Question 100 and Appendix). The National Cancer Institute (NCI) has a toll-free number (1-800-4-CANCER) where you can call to find a specialist in your area. You can also call the nearest university hospital to find a specialist.

   The American College of Surgeons' Web site (*www. facs.org*) lists its members by specialty. You can go to the "public information" tab and look for surgeons in your area with a specific specialty.

   The American Society of Clinical Oncology has a Web site, People Living with Cancer (*www.plwc.org*), where you can search for an oncologist, surgeon, or radiation oncologist in your area.
4. Make a list of a few possible choices in case you are not able to get an appointment within the time frame needed. Having a few choices for physicians will also enable you to get multiple treatment options so that you can make a well-informed decision.

After you have found a specific doctor, it is important to evaluate whether or not he or she is qualified. Important things to consider are:

- Credentials: Board certification in a specialty area ensures proficiency in that area. Residency or fellowship training at a major academic cancer center involves training under experts within the field of oncology. Basic information about the doctor's schooling and training can be found on the American

Medical Association's Physician Select Web site at *www.ama-assn.org/aps/amahg.htm.*
- Technical skills: For surgeons, it is pretty well established that high volume centers tend to have better outcomes than low volume surgical centers. It may be helpful to find out the number of stomach cancers seen by the practice.
- Hospital affiliation: Although comprehensive cancer centers and university hospitals generally have access to more technology and clinical trials, it is important to realize that the best treatment option for you may be close to home. The majority of cancer care in the U.S. is provided by community oncologists who generally do an excellent job with their cancer care.
- Compassion: You will want a physician who understands your fears and will discuss your concerns. It is hard to ascertain this on the first meeting, so you should go with your "gut" feeling.
- Approachability: You should feel comfortable asking your physician questions about the disease and your cancer care. A physician who is not approachable will only add to your anxiety.

Beware of physicians who promise a cancer cure. Truthfully, the best we can do is give you an estimate of the odds. Generally speaking, the smaller and more localized the cancer, the better the prognosis. With cancers that have metastasized, our aim is to control the disease.

Jim's comment:

I think finding the right team of medical experts is by far the most important thing you will ever do to ensure your chances for survival. Statistics say that patient survival rates are highest in major cancer centers. You might think you are better off getting individual care by someone only seeing a few patients, but that is the very thing a large cancer center has over other facilities. Ask your doctor how many patients he or she treats every day with your type of cancer. Ask what the success rates have been. Make a list of the questions you want to ask, and make sure you ask the same questions to all the doctors. The answers will make your choice more obvious. Don't start any treatments until you are very comfortable with the cancer center and the doctors that will be taking care of you.

Ann's comment:

Making a decision about where to be treated for the cancer was extraordinarily difficult and stressful. I was diagnosed at a very good hospital where I had been treated for another illness for over two years. Since I wanted a second opinion, a colleague at work put me in touch with a woman who works at a cancer center near where I live, and she helped me get an appointment there with a surgeon who specializes in gastric cancer. I knew I needed surgery as quickly as possible, and I had to decide where to go. I felt torn because I was familiar with the gastroenterology staff at the first hospital, and it was just four blocks from my apartment. But the second institution was devoted exclusively to cancer care, and had an international reputation. I agonized for days, seeking opinions from family members and other doctors who had treated me for other ailments. In the end, I listened to my family, including my mother, who was treated at the cancer center more than 30 years ago. Looking back, I'm so glad I went with the cancer center because I think the team that treated me had far more cumulative experience with cancer patients than the doctors I would have seen at the first hospital.

27. Who are the members of the health care team? What does interdisciplinary mean?

Your health care team may include physicians (medical oncologist, radiation oncologist, and/or surgeon), nurses, pharmacists, social workers, psychiatrists, psychologists, and nutrition specialists.

- *Medical oncologists* are board certified internists who choose to acquire additional education and training to subspecialize in medical oncology. They specialize in the use of medical and chemotherapeutic treatments for cancer. They manage the cancer patient through all phases of care.
- *Surgeons* are doctors who have completed at least five years of highly specialized training after medical school to gain the skills necessary to be called a "surgeon." If your cancer is operable, you would be referred to a surgeon to have the disease removed surgically. A surgical oncologist is one who specializes in performing cancer surgery. Surgical oncologists are also board certified and are experts in performing adequate operations on cancer, for example, operations with wide surgical margins and adequate dissection and removal of regional lymph nodes to ensure removal of all sites of regional disease.
- *Radiation oncologists* are physicians who have been trained to treat cancer with radiation.
- *Gastroenterologists* are physicians who specialize in the diagnosis and treatment of gastrointestinal diseases.
- *Pathologists* are physicians trained to examine and evaluate tissues and cells. The pathologist looks at the biopsy tissue and prepares a report for the oncologist or surgeon.
- *Nurses* play an important role in your health care team and are usually in charge of actually implementing the plan of care that your doctor has set up. This includes the administration of medications, monitoring and triaging the side effects of your medications and treatment, assisting with insurance and payment problems, and helping with the psychosocial needs of the patient and caregiver. Nurses also assist you with completing the paperwork to receive social service assistance and government and/or private disability benefits.
- *Pharmacists* are licensed professionals who distribute medications and chemotherapy treatments prescribed by your oncologist and other health practitioners. They

provide information to patients about medications and their use. They advise physicians and other health practitioners on the selection, dosages, interactions, and side effects of medications. Pharmacists also monitor the health and progress of patients in response to drug therapy to ensure the safe and effective use of medication.

- *Social workers* are professionally trained in counseling and practical assistance. They provide the broadest range of help to assist with counseling and finding support groups for you and/or your family. They also assist with helping to locate services in your community.
- *Psychiatrists* are medical doctors who specialize in providing psychotherapy or general psychological help. They can prescribe medications for patients who are depressed, anxious, or otherwise unable to cope psychologically as a result of a new cancer diagnosis or a preexisting condition that has been exacerbated by a cancer diagnosis.
- *Psychologists* are not medical doctors, but they have obtained a doctoral degree in psychology and counseling. They are able to assist with counseling services to cancer patients who are depressed, anxious, or unhappy and having a difficult time coping with a new diagnosis.
- *Nutrition specialists* can suggest ways to get enough calories, vitamins, and nutrition to help a patient feel better and control his or her weight. They can give tips about increasing appetite if a patient experiences nausea, heartburn, or fatigue as a result of illness or treatment.

Interdisciplinary care occurs when a range of disciplines (including physicians, nurses, social workers, and pharmacists) work together as a team at one facility to provide your health care. This approach to care has several advantages, including fewer trips to the doctor, less time from diagnosis to start of treatment, and efficient high-quality care.

Interdisciplinary care

A range of disciplines (doctors, nurses, social workers, pharmacists, and others) working together as a team at one facility to provide your health care.

28. Should I get a second opinion?

Before you and your doctor decide on a treatment, you may want to get a **second opinion**. A second opinion is often a good way to make sure that you are receiving the best possible care. It is important to have confidence in your doctor's recommendations and if you are having doubts, a second opinion may give you reassurance. It can also give you the peace of mind knowing that you have explored all your options. However, be aware of the possibility that the second opinion may also give you conflicting recommendations, which may cause significant anxiety. You may be able to find the right choice for you by asking more questions and going with the answers that make the most sense to you. Some patients worry that this may offend their doctor. My advice is not to worry about this—it is your right to seek the advice of a second opinion. Many insurance companies will cover a second opinion if your doctor requests it. It is usually not a problem to take several weeks to get a second opinion, and in most cases, the delay in treatment will not make the treatment less effective. However, too many second opinions may result in unacceptable delays in therapy. You should discuss this delay with your physician so that he/she can decide whether treatment needs to be started right away. Your doctor may refer you to one or more specialists. At cancer centers, several specialists often work together as a team.

There are a number of ways to find a physician for a second opinion.

There are a number of ways to find a physician for a second opinion. You can call the NCI's Cancer Information Service at 1-800-4-Cancer. You can contact a local or state medical society or nearby hospital that can provide you with the names of specialists. The American Board of Medical Specialties also has a list of doctors who have received training and passed boards in a particular specialty. This directory can be found in most public libraries.

29. How do I emotionally handle a new cancer diagnosis?

Of the many health problems that can occur, being diagnosed with cancer is among the most feared. Having a cancer diagnosis and undergoing treatment for the cancer will change your life and your outlook on life. There are many support systems available to you and several things you can do to help cope with the diagnosis.

- Allow yourself to experience the full range of emotions (anger, fear, denial, anxiety, and depression).
- Educate yourself about your specific diagnosis (use the Internet as a resource, but always remember that the information may not be 100% accurate). Knowledge is power: the more you know about your cancer and its treatment, the better equipped you will be at handling what comes your way.
- Allow your family and friends to be a support system. Don't believe that you have to handle this alone.

Having a cancer diagnosis and undergoing treatment for the cancer will change your life and your outlook on life. There are many support systems available to you and several things you can do to help cope with the diagnosis.

Jim's comment:

I had a father who died of lung cancer, but of course, he smoked, and I have never had a cigarette touch my lips. My mother died of ovarian cancer and I surely didn't need to worry about that as a man. WRONG! It appears I had all the signs for a propensity of cancer in my family, I just didn't know. My wife and caregiver never let me believe there was a chance we would not survive. My children immediately gathered around me and offered love and support. My friends from my childhood, college, and adult life prayed for me constantly and were always there to support me through the treatments and after. I give thanks to all of them.

Ann's comment:

Soon after my diagnosis and surgery, I started looking into complementary and alternative therapies and support groups. I made an appointment with a psychiatrist at the cancer center where I was treated and got a prescription for the anti-anxiety medication Ativan. In addition, my surgeon wrote me a prescription for Ambien, the sleep aid. I'd never taken anti-anxiety medication or sleeping pills before but decided I needed them in my self-help arsenal in case I had problems. I also looked into massage, acupuncture, meditation, and psychotherapy. But from the time I was diagnosed in June until the end of my chemo and radiation in late November, I had little time or energy for any kind of supplemental therapy. I was just focused on getting through the treatment. It was only when the medical treatment was over and I was starting to feel better physically that I finally started to deal with the psychological aspects of the disease. Even though it's been 2 ½ years since my diagnosis, I feel as though I'm only just now starting to get a grip on the anxiety about the cancer. I've been participating in a support group with other cancer survivors and trying to fit daily meditation into my routine. I work out with a trainer at my gym a couple times a week and try to exercise as much as possible. When all else fails, I take Ativan to quiet my racing mind.

30. Is depression a possibility?

A certain degree of depression is common in people who are coping with cancer. But when a person has long-lasting emotional distress or is unable or unwilling to carry out normal daily activities, that person may have clinical depression. In fact, about 25% of people with cancer experience clinical depression, according to the American Cancer Society, causing distress, impaired functioning, and decreased ability to follow a treatment schedule. Caregivers should be alert for symptoms of depression. If you notice symptoms of depression, you should help the patient to seek assistance from a health care professional. Clinical depression can be managed with a variety of treatments including medication, psychotherapy, a combination of both, or some other specialized treatment. These therapies can improve the quality of life and psychological condition of people with cancer.

31. What is clinical depression?

Depression is a disease. There are many signs of depression that include:

- Feeling sad or "down" most of the time
- Having a loss of interest in daily activities
- Unexplained weight loss (without dieting) or weight gain
- Feeling slowed down, restless, or agitated on a daily basis—enough that other people notice
- Feeling that you would be "better off dead" and considering the idea of killing yourself, or actually making a suicide attempt
- Having trouble concentrating, remembering, or making decisions that would have been routine under normal circumstances
- Having no energy, feeling wasted
- Having trouble sleeping or waking early in the morning; sleeping too much
- Feelings of guilt, helplessness, and worthlessness

Having five or more of these symptoms for more than a few weeks in a row is a worrisome sign of clinical depression. However, for the cancer patient, many of these signs are considered normal effects of the cancer or its treatment. For example, cancer and its treatment with chemotherapy may result in anemia, which in turn may cause fatigue. Chemotherapy can cause difficulty with concentration or remembering, or with making decisions. Furthermore, it is natural to feel sad, grieve, and be depressed after being diagnosed with cancer (see Question 30). If these signs and symptoms continue, ask your doctor or a qualified health or mental health professional for assistance in distinguishing clinical depression from a normal reaction to the diagnosis of cancer.

Depression

A medical condition in which the person suffering feels an intractable sense of loss or helplessness. Situational depression occurs as a result or consequence of a particular event or circumstance that occured.

It is natural to feel sad, grieve, and be depressed after being diagnosed with cancer. If these signs and symptoms continue, ask your doctor or a qualified health or mental health professional for assistance in distinguishing clinical depression from a normal reaction to the diagnosis of cancer.

32. What questions do I ask my health care team?

Always remember to write down key concerns and a list of questions before going to your appointments with members of your health care team. Some common questions include:

- What type of cancer do I have?
- What is the stage of cancer? Is there any evidence that the cancer has spread?
- What is the recommended treatment for my disease and why? Are there other treatment options?
- How often is my treatment, and how long will it take?
- When and why should I call the doctor's office?
- How will we know whether the treatment is working?
- What should I do to be ready for treatment?
- Based on what you've learned about my cancer, what is my prognosis (the outlook for survival)?
- What is the goal of my treatment—to cure or to ease symptoms?
- If I am to have surgery, what is your experience in this type of surgery for stomach cancer?
- If I am to have surgery, what is the experience of the hospital in this type of surgery for stomach cancer?
- Could you recommend a social worker, psychotherapist, or support group for me (or my family members)?

If necessary, ask for medications to help you through your psychosocial issues (antidepressants, anti-anxiety medicine, and/or sleeping medications). It is important to remember that the stress of dealing with your diagnosis can cause mood changes, and that the treatments and medications you receive may also cause some alterations in your mood.

Acknowledge your fear and anxiety. It is normal to have these feelings, and it is also essential to discuss these feelings with your health care team, family, and friends. You should utilize these people to help you navigate through your new diagnosis and treatment.

Ask your health care team all the questions that you have. Educating yourself about your disease is the best way to know what to expect, and this in turn gives you some power in an otherwise powerless situation. In fact, powerlessness is a common complaint of cancer patients, who feel they have no power over the disease, treatment, or its side effects. So it is essential to maintain control whenever you can. Be an active partner in your care, discuss your needs with your doctor, and help formulate your treatment plan.

Jim's comment:

I agree that you can never ask enough questions, but you will soon learn that you don't even know the correct questions to ask. But with time they will become clear and you will ask them. I highly recommend reading and talking with others with your specific type of cancer. I always found it very helpful, and I think the people offering the advice or comments were glad to be of help and support.

Ann's comment:

From the day I was diagnosed, I made lists of questions to ask the doctors and nurses. I would bring those lists to my appointments, but often it was very hard to concentrate on the answers to the questions. That's why I always went with another person—usually my husband, but sometimes a relative. When we compared notes afterwards, it always surprised me what I didn't hear. Although I tried to be thorough and prepare for the appointments, I had to force myself to go through the lists of questions. Sometimes I felt that the doctor was in a hurry. I didn't want to be a "pain in the butt" kind of patient and take up too much of the doctor's time. Moreover, I wanted him or her to like me. But I had friends and relatives who encouraged me to speak up for myself, even if I felt that I was being annoying. In reality, no one was ever less than professional in responding to my questions, and eventually going to the appointments became easier.

PART FIVE

Treatment Options

How is stomach cancer treated?

What long term effects should I know about following the removal of my stomach?

How does my doctor know if my treatment is working? What if my treatment doesn't work?

More . . .

33. How is stomach cancer treated?

Stomach cancer can be treated in a variety of ways. The most common treatments include surgery, chemotherapy, and radiation therapy. These treatments may be used alone or in combination with one another to optimize response.

Surgery

Surgery is the primary mode of treatment for localized cancer.

Surgery is the primary mode of treatment for localized cancer. The following types of surgery for localized cancer may be used:

- *Subtotal gastrectomy.* Removal of the part of the stomach that contains cancer, nearby lymph nodes, and parts of other tissues and organs near the tumor. The spleen may be removed. The spleen is an organ in the upper abdomen that filters the blood and removes old blood cells.
- *Total gastrectomy.* Removal of the entire stomach, nearby lymph nodes, as well as parts of the esophagus, small intestine, and other tissues near the tumor. The spleen may be removed. The esophagus is connected to the small intestine so the patient can continue to eat and swallow.

If the tumor is blocking the opening to the stomach but the cancer cannot be completely removed by standard surgery, the following procedures may be used:

Endoluminal stent placement

A procedure to insert a stent (a thin, expandable tube) in order to keep a passage (such as arteries or the esophagus) open.

Endoscopic laser surgery

A procedure in which an endoscope (a thin, lighted tube) with a laser attached is inserted into the body.

Chemotherapy

A type of treatment for cancer that uses drugs to stop the growth of cancer cells, either by killing the cells or by stopping them from dividing.

- *Endoluminal stent placement.* A procedure to insert a stent (a thin, expandable tube) in order to keep a passage (such as arteries or the esophagus) open. For tumors blocking the opening to the stomach, surgery may be done to place a stent from the esophagus to the stomach to allow the patient to eat normally.
- *Endoscopic laser surgery.* A procedure in which an endoscope (a thin, lighted tube) with a laser attached is inserted into the body. A laser is an intense beam of light that can be used as a knife.

- *Electrocautery.* A procedure that uses an electrical current to create heat. This is sometimes used to remove lesions or control bleeding.

Chemotherapy

Chemotherapy is a type of treatment for cancer that uses drugs to stop the growth of cancer cells, either by killing the cells or by stopping them from dividing. When chemotherapy is taken by mouth or injected into a vein or muscle, the drugs enter the bloodstream and can reach cancer cells throughout the body via blood circulation, called **systemic chemotherapy**. When chemotherapy is placed directly into the spinal column, an organ, or a body cavity such as the abdomen, the drugs mainly affect cancer cells in those areas, called **regional chemotherapy**. The method of administering the chemotherapy depends on the type and stage of cancer being treated. For stomach cancer, the current standard is that chemotherapy is given via the bloodstream as systemic therapy. At this time, regional chemotherapy is considered experimental for the treatment of stomach cancer.

Chemotherapy is the treatment of choice for metastatic stomach cancer. There are many types of drugs and each has its own side effects (see Questions 44–60).

Radiation therapy

Radiation therapy is a type of cancer treatment that uses high-energy x-rays or other types of radiation to kill cancer cells or keep them from growing. There are two types of radiation therapy. **External radiation therapy** uses a machine outside the body to send radiation toward the cancer. **Internal radiation therapy** uses a radioactive substance sealed in needles, seeds, wires, or catheters placed directly into or near the cancer. The way the radiation therapy is given depends on the type and stage of cancer being treated.

For cancer of the stomach and gastroesophageal junction, radiation is almost always given with chemotherapy for

Systemic chemotherapy

Chemotherapy that is injected into a muscle or vein and subsequently enters the bloodstream. The chemotherapy reaches cancer cells via blood circulation.

Regional chemotherapy

Chemotherapy that is placed directly into the spinal column, organ, or body cavity to affect cells in a certain region or area.

Radiation therapy

A type of cancer treatment that uses high-energy x-rays or other types of radiation to kill cancer cells or keep them from growing.

External radiation therapy

Radiation treatment that uses an external radiation source that is then directed or aimed at a specific position within the body.

Internal radiation therapy

Radiation treatment that uses a source that can be directly injected or inserted into a specific position within the body.

Treatment Options

localized disease (see next section). For metastatic disease, radiation may be given by external beam to control symptoms of pain or to improve swallowing.

Chemoradiation

Chemoradiation
Treatment that combines chemotherapy with radiation therapy.

Adjuvant therapy
Therapy to treat cancer that is given after surgery.

Neoadjuvant therapy
Therapy to treat cancer that is given before surgery.

Chemoradiation combines chemotherapy and radiation therapy to increase the effects of both. Chemoradiation treatment given after surgery to increase the chances of a cure is called **adjuvant therapy**. If chemoradiation treatment is given before surgery, it is called **neoadjuvant therapy**. Adjuvant therapy is therapy given following surgery.

For stomach cancer, chemoradiation therapy is commonly given following surgical resection for localized disease. This type of radiation is external radiation, or external beam radiation. Chemoradiation is also given before or instead of surgery for cancers of the gastroesophageal junction (see Question 39).

Biologic therapy

Biologic therapy
A treatment that uses the patient's immune system to fight cancer.

Immune system
A collection of mechanisms that protects against infection by identifying and killing pathogens.

Biologic therapy, also called *biotherapy* or *immunotherapy*, is a treatment that uses the patient's **immune system** to fight cancer. Substances made by the body or made in a laboratory are used to boost, direct, or restore the body's natural defenses against cancer. Although this therapy is not generally effective in the treatment of stomach cancer, research is ongoing and there is hope for more use of this therapy in the future.

34. How do we decide what treatment options are best for me?

There are several factors that play a role in deciding the best treatment for you. These factors include the location of the tumor (gastroesophageal junction versus stomach), the extent of the tumor (localized or metastatic), and your personal health status (for example, whether you have other medical problems that may make treatment—surgery or chemotherapy—dangerous). Your cancer specialist will take each of these into consideration when creating a treatment plan for you. Often, the best treatment requires the coordination of several subspecialties, such as surgical oncology, medical oncology, and radiation oncology, to devise the best and most comprehensive treatment plan for you.

35. What are the various approaches for the treatment of localized gastroesophageal (GEJ) cancer?

As described in Part 1, the gastroesophageal junction is the junction between the stomach and the esophagus. Cancers of the GEJ that have spread beyond the primary area and have metastasized are treated with chemotherapy, just as if they are metastatic stomach cancer. However, localized GEJ cancers—by virtue of its location between the esophagus and stomach—are sometimes treated like cancers of the esophagus and sometimes treated like cancers of the stomach. The treatment options available for localized GEJ cancer include the following:

- chemotherapy followed by surgery
- chemotherapy with radiation, either with or without surgery
- surgery alone
- surgery followed by chemotherapy with radiation
- photodynamic therapy (light therapy to kill superficial cancers) for very early stage cancers (see Question 36).

For very early stage GEJ cancers, treatment is often surgery alone (see Question 36). For localized GEJ cancer that has spread deeper into the wall of the gastroesophageal junction or to local lymph nodes, the choice of treatment plan is made based upon a variety of factors, including how much of the cancer has gone into the esophagus or how much of the cancer has gone into the stomach. Cancers that are in the GEJ and extend into the esophagus are more commonly treated like esophagus cancer. This means they are more likely given

Treatment Options

Cancers of the GEJ that have spread beyond the primary area and have metastasized are treated with chemotherapy, just as if they are metastatic stomach cancer.

For localized GEJ cancer that has spread deeper into the wall of the gastroesophageal junction or to local lymph nodes, the choice of treatment plan is made based upon a variety of factors, including how much of the cancer has gone into the esophagus or how much of the cancer has gone into the stomach.

chemotherapy with radiation, sometimes followed by surgery. Alternatively, GEJ cancers that extend into the stomach are commonly treated like localized stomach cancer—that is, chemotherapy followed by and given after surgery, or surgery first followed by chemotherapy and radiation.

Your underlying health also factors into the decision process. For example, if you have heart or lung disease, you may not be well enough to undergo a rigorous operation on your stomach and GEJ. In this case, chemotherapy and radiation may be the best treatment option because then you may not require surgery.

Jim's comment:

I was diagnosed with adenocarcinoma of the GEJ and it was staged at T3N1. My protocol included chemotherapy, followed by chemo and radiation, and culminated with surgery. Part of my esophagus and part of my stomach were removed.

36. What is the best treatment for early stage GEJ cancer?

For the earliest stage cancers of the GEJ, surgery is considered the best option. Surgery on the GEJ can be performed by removing the lower part of the esophagus, by removing the stomach, or by removing both. During this surgery, the surgeon will remove part of the lower esophagus and part of the stomach to ensure complete removal of the cancer. This is what is meant by a "wide surgical margin." The surgeon will then need to reconnect the remaining stomach with the remaining esophagus. This is called the anastomosis. For esophagus cancer, where more of the esophagus is required to come out, the stomach may not be long enough to make a good anastomosis. In this case, a piece of the colon may be used as a bridge between the esophagus and stomach—that is, a new esophagus is made. This type of surgery is considered major surgery, and you should plan to be in the hospital for 1 to 2 weeks. It is best to have this surgery done by an experienced surgeon who has special training in thoracic or gastrointestinal surgery. Recent research has shown that this type of surgery is safer and associated with fewer complications when done at a high-volume center, one that performs this surgery often.

For patients who are not able to have surgery or who may have very early stage GEJ cancer (just into the first layer of the intestinal wall), **photodynamic therapy** may be an option. Photodynamic therapy is a type of light or laser treatment. First, a chemical called photofrin (porfimer sodium) is injected into the area where the cancer is via an endoscope. This chemical, the photofrin, makes the cancer cells sensitive to the high-energy light that is directed on them through the endoscope. When exposed to high-energy laser light by the endoscope, the cells that have taken up the photofrin are destroyed. The timing of when the laser light is directed through the endoscope to the cells is critical for maximal cell killing. The high-energy laser light is directed at the cells when the photofrin is concentrated in the cancer cells and not in the normal cells. This treatment is approved by the FDA (Food and Drug Administration) in the United States for the treatment of early-staged cancer. The problem with this type of therapy is that it only works as far as the laser light can penetrate. For cancers that are still early stage and penetrate into the esophagus more than a few millimeters, photodynamic therapy may not be the best option. In this case, surgery may be the best option. Photodynamic therapy is also approved as palliative treatment for cancers that grow close to the lumen of the GEJ.

Photodynamic therapy

High intensity light treatment using a chemical photosensitizer to make the cancer cells sensitive to the treatment.

For patients who are not able to have surgery or who may have very early stage GEJ cancer (just into the first layer of the intestinal wall), photodynamic therapy may be an option. Photodynamic therapy is a type of light or laser treatment.

37. When is chemoradiation used for the treatment of GEJ cancer?

For cancer of the GEJ that has penetrated deeper into the wall of the gastroesophageal junction or has involved lymph nodes, chemotherapy with radiation is often considered a good first option. The purpose of the chemotherapy when given with radiation is to make the radiation work better. Chemotherapy attacks cancer cells by attacking the cell-dividing machinery of the cell (see Questions 44 and 45). Radiation attacks cancer cells by high-energy radiation beams that damage DNA. By aiming the radiation beam directly at the area that has cancer, the cancer cells can be selectively killed. The combination of chemotherapy and radiation is a highly effective double attack on the cancer cell.

Combined chemotherapy and radiation should also be considered as the main treatment if the cancer is localized to the GEJ but is not able to be removed by surgery because of extension to nearby structures.

Several issues must be considered when planning chemotherapy with radiation in the treatment of localized GEJ cancer. First, with regard to chemotherapy, there are many active drugs that work particularly well with radiation. Historically, the chemotherapy drugs most commonly used in combination with radiation are fluorouracil and cisplatin. This treatment regimen is considered to be a standard option in combination with radiation. Other chemotherapy drugs that have good activity with radiation include taxanes (such as docetaxel) and irinotecan. Currently, there is less experience with these newer drugs in combination with radiation, but they are often used as substitutes because they have fewer side effects as compared to cisplatin and fluorouracil. For a full description of these drugs, see Question 44.

Second, with regard to radiation, it is important to plan the treatment very carefully. Your radiation oncologist will look at the films of your cancer and measure the cancer precisely. He or she will then map out the treatment field and create a mold of your body so that the radiation can be directed precisely to the tumor and surrounding tissue. Careful planning by an experienced radiation oncologist is critical for maximal tumor killing. Careful planning will also help minimize side effects resulting from radiation exposure to normal structures.

38. Do I need to have surgery after chemotherapy and radiation for localized GEJ cancer?

There is no clear-cut answer to this question at this time. We do know that for localized esophageal cancer, surgery alone and chemoradiation alone offer good treatment options that are both curative. The chance of success with both options is about the same. However, what is the value of having all three modalities of therapy: chemotherapy, radiation, and surgery? Recently, large studies were conducted to look at this question, and the answer is still not clear. These studies did not prove a survival benefit of surgery following chemoradiation or of chemoradiation preceding surgery. However, there may be a benefit in reducing the chance of a local recurrence at the GEJ if surgery is performed following chemotherapy with radiation.

In the United States, the usual treatment program would begin with chemotherapy and chemoradiation. It is reasonable to stop here, particularly if the risk of surgery is high, for example, if there is preexisting heart disease or lung disease that increases the chance of complications for surgery. If, however, there is still disease in the GEJ after all the treatment is given and the risk of surgery is minimal, proceeding with an operation is also reasonable.

Jim's comment:

I would have thought that after all my chemo and radiation, there was no way a cancer cell existed in my body, but how wrong I was. After my surgery, the biopsy came back on the dissected tissue and it still showed live cancer cells. This was proof to me that the surgery was essential.

39. What treatment options are best for localized stomach cancer based on staging?

The best treatment option for stomach cancer is always evolving. At this time, the best treatment option for early stage stomach cancer (stage 0 or I) is surgery (see summary that follows). Stage II and stage III stomach cancers are called locally advanced stomach cancers. For these cancers, there are two standard treatment options. One option is to proceed with surgery first and then, following recovery from surgery, proceed with chemotherapy and radiation. This is called **adjuvant chemoradiation** and is based on a national clinical trial in the United States that was published in 2001 in the *New England Journal of Medicine.* The other option for stages II and III stomach cancers is to proceed with chemotherapy first, followed by surgery, and then more chemotherapy. This treatment is based on a large clinical trial performed in England and published in the *New England Journal of Medicine* in 2006. Here is a summary of the treatment options based on stage of cancer:

Adjuvant chemoradiation

Chemotherapy and radiation given following curative intent surgery for locally advanced gastric or GEJ carcinomas.

Stage 0 Gastric Cancer (Carcinoma in Situ)

Treatment of stage 0 gastric cancer is usually surgery (total or subtotal gastrectomy).

Stage I Gastric Cancer

Treatment of stage I gastric cancer may include the following:

- Surgery (total or subtotal gastrectomy).
- Surgery (total or subtotal gastrectomy) followed by chemoradiation therapy. This option is sometimes considered if the cancer involves lymph nodes (e.g., T1N1 cancers).

Stage II Gastric Cancer

Treatment of stage II gastric cancer may include the following:

- Surgery (total or subtotal gastrectomy). This option is really only considered if the patient is not well enough to receive any further therapy.
- Surgery (total or subtotal gastrectomy) followed by chemoradiation therapy.
- Chemotherapy given before and after surgery.

Stage III Gastric Cancer

Treatment of stage III gastric cancer may include the following:

- Surgery (total or subtotal gastrectomy). This option is really only considered if the patient is not well enough to receive any further therapy.
- Surgery followed by chemoradiation therapy.
- Chemotherapy given before and after surgery.

For stages II and III stomach cancers, it is sometimes not easy to choose between starting off with chemotherapy and starting off with surgery. Our bias is to start with chemotherapy first, based on these reasons:

1. Patients tend to tolerate chemotherapy better if given before the surgery on their stomach.
2. Sometimes after surgery, patients may not heal well enough and fast enough to begin treatment within a reasonable amount of time, in which case the benefit of adjuvant treatment that is delayed is not clear. On the other hand, some physicians and patients may be concerned about the cancer growing while on chemotherapy. Fortunately, however, this occurs rarely and may have prevented a surgery that would not have been of any benefit.

For stages II and III stomach cancers, it is sometimes not easy to choose between starting off with chemotherapy and starting off with surgery.

40. How do I prepare for surgery?

The best way to prepare for a surgical procedure is to be in the best physical shape possible. Surgery is physically draining

Keeping a positive attitude and taking time for yourself are ways to help keep your mind at peace. Some patients find it helpful to speak to someone who has undergone the same surgery and is now fully recovered. Many hospitals have patient-to-patient volunteer programs that assist in this communication.

on the body. You should develop and maintain a program of activity throughout your course of treatment. Simple things like walking 15 to 20 minutes a day will help your body stay fit for surgery.

Mental well-being is just as important as physical well-being when it comes to surgery. Keeping a positive attitude and taking time for yourself are ways to help keep your mind at peace. Some patients find it helpful to speak to someone who has undergone the same surgery and is now fully recovered. Many hospitals have patient-to-patient volunteer programs that assist in this communication.

41. Can I live without a stomach?

Yes! You can lead a long, normal life with just a partial stomach or without the entire stomach. In the event that you need to have some or all of your stomach removed, you should be aware of the following concerns. It may be hard to gain weight, or you may find you are always losing weight. You may find that you have to watch what you eat to avoid symptoms of flushing and diarrhea following your meals. You may feel tired from being anemic; the drop in blood counts can come from low levels of iron or vitamin B_{12}. Finally, you may not absorb calcium very well and may be prone to reduced bone mineral density. However, with careful monitoring, there is no reason why you cannot live your normal lifespan after having stomach cancer surgery.

Dumping syndrome

A group of symptoms that occur when food or liquid enters the small intestine too rapidly. These symptoms include cramps, nausea, diarrhea, and dizziness.

Another common problem after stomach surgery is **dumping syndrome** (see Question 42). This problem occurs when food or liquid enters the small intestine too fast. It can cause cramps, nausea, bloating, diarrhea, and dizziness. Eating smaller meals can help prevent dumping syndrome. During your meal, eat protein first, then fruits and vegetables, and then whole grains. The diet should be high in protein and low in carbohydrates. Drink 6 to 8 ounces of water per day to prevent dehydration and constipation. Drink slowly and not all at once. Do not drink with meals, and resume drinking one hour after meals. Eat three small dense meals and one high-protein supplement or snack each day. Also, you may wish to cut down on very sweet foods and drinks such as cookies, candy, soda, and juices. A registered dietitian or nutritionist can suggest foods to try. Also, your health care team may suggest medicine to control the symptoms.

You may need to take daily supplements of vitamins and minerals, such as calcium. You also may need injections of vitamin B_{12}.

Jim's comment:

Eating is totally different for me in some ways, and in other ways it is just the same. Yes, my stomach is half the size it was; and, yes, my doctors told me to eat six small meals a day. In the beginning, I didn't want to eat at all, but my weight started dropping and my wife told me we hadn't come this far for me to starve to death. So I began eating again. I have basically the same breakfast I have always had, but now I follow it with a small snack around 10:00 and then I eat my usual lunch, but only one glass of tea instead of my usual jumbo glass with refills. Again in the afternoon, I snack at 2:00 and 4:00, and then I have a normal dinner at 6:00 or 6:30. I had the wonderful occasion at a medical conference to go out to a steak house with my surgeon. He was thrilled to see one of his patients eat so normally and eat an entire filet. I was very thankful that he had made that a reality. Some foods that I used to say were my favorites no longer interest me, and other foods that I did not eat a lot of have now become my favorites.

Ann's comment:

I had two-thirds of my stomach removed, and it's amazing to me how much I can still eat. If I'm not careful, I could easily weigh more than my ideal weight. There are some things I can't tolerate since the surgery: fried and spicy foods, and most raw fruits and vegetables. In addition, I often feel queasy if I eat super-sweet desserts, especially things made of chocolate. But it hasn't been much of a sacrifice giving up those things. The two hardest things have been giving up coffee, which tends to cause terrible GI problems, and training myself to eat smaller quantities. I spent most of my life eating hefty portions, especially at dinner. If I do that now, I feel extremely uncomfortable. The battle to give up coffee has been especially hard, since I love the taste and smell, and the way it makes me feel. I've sworn it off countless times, only to slip up and start drinking it again. Right now, I'm abstaining, and I like to think it's for good. I doubt I could have quit without my husband. When I would "fall off the wagon," he would get very upset—and rightly so, since he is the one who has to listen to my complaints and help me get through the gastric distress.

42. What long-term effects should I know about following the removal of my stomach?

Following gastric cancer surgery, a common complaint is an inability to gain weight. Weight loss can be seen in up to 60% of patients following stomach cancer surgery.

Weight loss/malnutrition: Following gastric cancer surgery, a common complaint is an inability to gain weight. Weight loss can be seen in up to 60% of patients following stomach cancer surgery. One of the most important functions of the stomach is to act as a reservoir for food that you eat during a meal. Without a stomach, or with only a partial stomach, this reservoir is greatly diminished. Thus, your body may signal that you are full well before completing a normal-sized meal. The biggest challenge is to retrain your body to eat more frequent, smaller meals to maintain your weight. It is even more difficult to regain weight that was lost following surgery.

Dumping syndrome: Another common complaint is dumping syndrome (see Question 41). There are two parts to this syndrome: the first part being early symptoms, and the second part being late symptoms. Early symptoms of dumping syndrome begin 15 to 30 minutes after meals and consist of abdominal discomfort (cramps), nausea, diarrhea, belching, heart palpitations, sweating, light-headedness, and even rarely losing consciousness. These signs and symptoms are caused by the very rapid emptying of partially digested food into the small intestine, resulting in a shift of fluid to the intestines and a short-lived loss of fluid from the vascular space. The shift of fluid can then sometimes activate the intestines very quickly, causing the release of gastrointestinal hormones, and result in diarrhea 20 to 45 minutes following the meal. Late symptoms of dumping typically occur 90 minutes to 3 hours after a meal. Patients feel light-headed, weak, have sweats, and rarely can have loss of consciousness. This phase of dumping syndrome may be caused by a short-lived drop in the blood sugars due to the overcompensated release of insulin in response to the first phase of dumping. Dumping syndrome tends to be activated by foods rich in carbohydrates, especially sucrose (for example, corn syrup), and the best way to manage this is by dietary modification. Dumping also can be provoked by overeating and consuming liquids with meals. There have also been reports of symptoms after the ingestion of foods that are high in fat. Limit your fat intake because it can also lead to nausea and weight gain. Foods to avoid include ice cream, chocolate milk, pudding, frozen yogurt, dried fruits, canned or frozen fruits in syrup, fruit juice, sugar-coated cereal, doughnuts, cake, pies, cookies, soft drinks, table sugar, honey, candy, jams, jellies, syrup, fruit drinks, and lemonade. Eating slowly, taking a half hour for each meal, and chewing thoroughly will help alleviate these symptoms. Symptoms generally improve with time. Being cautious of the foods you eat will help minimize symptoms of dumping.

Anemia/Vitamin B$_{12}$ loss: One of the functions of the stomach is to help absorb vitamin B$_{12}$. The parietal cells of the stomach secrete a protein called intrinsic factor (as discussed earlier) that binds to this vitamin and help its absorption in the small intestines. Following stomach surgery, there may be reduced levels of vitamin B$_{12}$ being absorbed and measured in the blood because of a lack of intrinsic factor. This can be remedied with vitamin B$_{12}$ supplementation, most commonly given as an injection into the muscle once a month.

Many patients are also anemic from a decrease in iron storage. This is felt to be the result of malabsorption of iron in patients following stomach cancer surgery, either due to not eating well or reduced absorption in the stomach.

Loss of bone mineral density: Following stomach cancer surgery, a person may not absorb vitamin D and calcium well, resulting in loss of bone density, or osteoporosis. This results in softening of the bone, pain, weakness, and increased fragility, known as osteomalacia. Osteomalacia can occur in as many as 25% of patients following a partial resection of the stomach. It may take years before x-ray findings show reduced bone density. Bone fractures occur twice as commonly in men after gastric surgery as in a control population. Careful monitoring, including measurements of vitamin D and calcium, are important, especially in women. Supplementation of vitamin D and calcium can rectify this problem.

Bile acid reflux: You may have symptoms of heartburn accompanied by nausea and chest discomfort. If you were to have an upper endoscopy, mild inflammation and irritation of the surface of the remaining stomach or esophagus may result. This is caused by the reflux (reverse flow) of bile acids.

Jim's comment:

I was diagnosed because of my anemia, and I remain anemic. My levels are higher, but it appears to be one of the things I will just deal with for the rest of my life. The first time you ever experience dumping, you will definitely want to find out what caused it because you will never want to experience it again. In talking with other survivors, different things cause the dumping, and once you identify your specific causes, you will learn to avoid them.

43. What is the best treatment for metastatic stomach or GEJ cancer?

For stage IV stomach or GEJ cancer, the treatment of choice is chemotherapy. In the 1990s, four separate clinical trials were performed in Europe that compared giving chemotherapy versus not giving chemotherapy for metastatic stomach cancer. Each of the studies showed that the patients who were randomized to receive chemotherapy lived longer, and in at least one study, patients who received chemotherapy also had a better quality of life. There are many types of chemotherapy drugs available for stomach and GEJ cancers, and the field is ever evolving.

44. How does chemotherapy work?

Chemotherapy is a type of medication that is given to attack cancer cells. There are many different types of chemotherapy. Traditional chemotherapy attacks cells that are rapidly dividing, like most cancer cells. Because cancer cells tend to divide more frequently and without restraint, chemotherapy prefers to attack cancer cells rather than other cells in the body that divide less frequently. However, there are some normal cells that also divide rapidly, and these cells would be damaged by traditional chemotherapeutic agents. For example, cells of the small and large intestine often divide rapidly. When chemotherapy is administered, these cells may be damaged, resulting in nausea, vomiting, and diarrhea. In addition, the cells of the bone marrow divide rapidly to make new white and red blood cells. Once again, chemotherapy, by virtue of attacking rapidly dividing cells preferentially, can often cause a drop in the white and red blood cell counts as a result of killing these actively dividing normal cells.

Most cancer cells divide rapidly. Chemotherapy frequently attacks these dividing cells in different ways. Some chemotherapy drugs attack DNA replication, so that the cells cannot replicate adequately. Some chemotherapy drugs attack the DNA repair process. Some drugs attack microtubules,

There are many types of chemotherapy drugs available for stomach and GEJ cancers, and the field is ever evolving.

Chemotherapy, by virtue of attacking rapidly dividing cells preferentially, can often cause a drop in the white and red blood cell counts as a result of killing these actively dividing normal cells.

structures in the cell that allow for daughter cells to separate from the parent cell. Even though each class of chemotherapy agents may attack different portions of the cell machinery involved in the synthesis of DNA and cell division, the net effect and goal of the treatment is to kill those rapidly dividing cells. Because many of the drugs act differently on the cell division machinery, they can be combined in ways to maximize cell killing. This is the basis for giving combination chemotherapy (two or more drugs given simultaneously). However, the more drugs that are given together, the more side effects you may experience.

45. What are some active drugs in the treatment of stomach cancer?

Table 2 lists the classes of chemotherapy drugs that are active in the treatment of stomach cancer. The first and most commonly used drugs belong to a class called **Antimetabolites**. Fluorouracil is the most commonly used antimetabolite for the treatment of stomach cancer. Part of the process of cell division is to make a daughter copy that is identical to the cell's DNA. Thymidylate synthase is a critical cellular protein required in the synthesis of new DNA. Fluorouracil is the cornerstone of the standard treatment regimen for this disease. More recently, newer and more convenient drugs in this class have been tested and have been shown to be about equal in efficacy to fluorouracil. These drugs, capecitabine and S-1, are pills that are taken orally. Because these drugs can be taken at home, they are more appealing to patients and physicians compared to fluorouracil. The side effects of the drugs in this class are variable and commonly include diarrhea, nausea, vomiting, and mouth sores.

The **Heavy Metals**, also known as *platinum analogues*, are the next most commonly used class of agents in the treatment of stomach cancer. These drugs attack dividing cells by attacking the cell's DNA. They work by binding to the DNA and linking it together so that the cell cannot replicate its DNA.

Antimetabolites

A class of chemotherapy that inhibits DNA synthesis, often by inhibiting the enzyme thymidylate synthase.

Heavy Metals

Metal based anti-cancer drugs that kill by causing crosslinks in DNA strands.

Table 2   Classes of Chemotherapy Agents active in the treatment of stomach cancer.

Class	Agent	Mechanism of Action
Antibiotic	Mitomycin-C[1]	Produces interstrand DNA cross-links
Antimetabolite	5-Fluorouracil	Inhibits thymidylate synthase
	Methotrexate[1]	Inhibits purine nucleotide and thymidylate synthesis
	Pemetrexed	Inhibits thymidylate synthase
	Capecitabine	Reduces thymidine production and competes with uridine triphosphate for incorporation into RNA
	S-1[2]	Inhibits thymidylate synthase and CDHP, and competes with uridine triphosphate for incorporation into RNA
Anthracycline	Doxorubicin Epirubicin	Intercalates into DNA and interacts with topoisomerase II
Heavy Metal	Cisplatin Carboplatin Oxaliplatin	Produces intrastrand and interstrand DNA cross-links
Taxanes	Docetaxel Paclitaxel	Binds to and stabilizes tubulin, inhibiting microtubule disassembly
Topoisomerase Inhibitors	Etoposide[1]	Binds to and inhibits topoisomerase II
	Irinotecan	Binds to and inhibits topoisomerase I

1. Not routinely used in the U.S.
2. Currently investigational outside of Japan

Cisplatin is the most commonly used drug in this class, although oxaliplatin may be a close equivalent to Cisplatin. Oxaliplatin (Eloxatin®, Sanofi-Aventis Inc.) may have fewer side effects associated with its use and is therefore an appealing substitute in certain situations. Carboplatin is probably not as active as oxaliplatin or cisplatin in the treatment of stomach cancer, but it is sometimes the best option based on a patient's health status. Common side effects of the heavy metals include nausea, vomiting, fatigue, and a drop in blood counts.

Taxanes

A new class of anticancer drug that attacks microtubules.

Taxanes are the newest and next most commonly used class of drugs in the treatment of stomach cancer. Taxanes kill dividing cells by inhibiting the function of microtubules, the proteins that help the DNA strands separate from each other during cell division. Docetaxel (Taxotere®, Sanofi-Aventis Inc.) has recently been approved for use in combination with cisplatin and fluorouracil for the first line treatment of stomach cancer in both the United States and in Europe. Common side effects of taxanes include a drop in blood counts, the development of an allergic reaction to the chemical the drug is mixed in, and numbness and tingling.

Anthracyclines

An older class of chemotherapy drugs derived from antibiotics.

The **Anthracyclines** are among the oldest class of chemotherapy agents available. Historically, Doxorubicin (Adriamycin®, Pharmacia & Upjohn) was commonly used in combination with fluorouracil and methotrexate or mitomycin-C as part of the FAMTX or FAM regimens. These regimens were considered as the standard of therapy in the 1980s and early 1990s, and are not commonly used today. Epirubicin (Ellence®, Farmorubicin®, Pfizer Inc.) is more commonly used today, in combination with fluorouracil and cisplatin, as part of the ECF regimen. This is an active regimen that is used both for patients with metastatic disease and for patients with localized disease. Common side effects of this class of drugs include nausea, vomiting, and damage to the heart.

Topoisomerase Inhibitors

A new class of chemotherapy that kills cancer cells by inhibiting an enzyme, topoisomerase I, involved in DNA repair.

The **Topoisomerase Inhibitors** form the last commonly used class of drugs in the treatment of stomach cancer. Irinotecan (Campto®, Sanofi-Aventis Inc.; Camptosar®, Pfizer Inc.) is active in the treatment of stomach cancer, particularly when given in combination with fluorouracil or cisplatin. Common side effects of this class of drugs include diarrhea and a drop in blood counts.

46. What recent clinical trial data support some of the newer chemotherapy regimens in the treatment of stomach cancer?

A recent analysis that combined several studies together confirmed that chemotherapy does provide a significant advantage in survival over not receiving chemotherapy. This study also suggested that combination treatment, in particular anthracyclines (e.g. epirubicin) combined with cisplatin and fluorouracil, was better than other therapies. Recently, there have also been several studies examining whether oxaliplatin and capecitabine can be substituted for cisplatin and fluorouracil, respectively. One such study performed in England involved about 1000 patients. The results of this study effectively demonstrate that oxaliplatin may be substituted for cisplatin, and that capecitabine may be substituted for fluorouracil when administered as a low dose continuous infusion. In the U.S., oxaliplatin is approved by the Center for Medicare and Medicaid Services (the governing body that approves drugs for Medicare and Medicaid) for the treatment of gastric cancer.

There are several clinical trials that show that docetaxel is useful in the treatment of stomach cancer. One important trial was a randomized study of docetaxel combined with cisplatin and fluorouracil compared to cisplatin and fluorouracil alone. The results of the trial showed that the patients who were randomly assigned to receive docetaxel in combination with cisplatin and fluorouracil had a slightly higher chance of having their cancer shrink and were able to continue treatment longer than patients who did not receive docetaxel. Most importantly, patients who received docetaxel along with cisplatin and fluorouracil lived slightly longer than patients who received only cisplatin and fluorouracil.

Based on this data, the United States Food and Drug Administration, as well as the governing body in Europe, the European Union, approved the use of docetaxel along with cisplatin and fluorouracil in the treatment of stomach and gastroesophageal junction adenocarcinoma.

The drawback to this study was that patients in both of the treatment arms, cisplatin and fluorouracil with or without docetaxel, experienced many side effects. Patients commonly had nausea, vomiting, fatigue, weakness, and a drop in their blood counts. Active research is ongoing to see how best to administer docetaxel in combination with cisplatin and fluorouracil so that patients can get the maximum benefit from drug therapy and tolerate treatment better to maximize their quality of life.

47. How do you choose which chemotherapy drug or combination to use?

Several different drugs are useful in the treatment of stomach cancer. Generally speaking, any single drug has modest activity and few side effects. Combinations of chemotherapy agents, particularly drugs from different classes, tend to be more effective against the cancer, but they may also have more side effects. In the treatment of stomach cancer, we try to use the best combination possible to maximize therapy. If the tumor starts to grow or spread, or when a new cancer spot develops, current treatment needs to be switched from one class of drugs to another class of drugs.

Combinations of chemotherapy agents, particularly drugs from different classes, tend to be more effective against the cancer, but they may also have more side effects. In the treatment of stomach cancer, we try to use the best combination possible to maximize therapy.

At this time, it is impossible to predict which class of drugs is the best to use first; this is an active area of research. However, for an otherwise healthy younger person with stomach cancer, cisplatin- and fluorouracil-based treatment would be considered standard. Based on the most recent clinical trial data, that would be the combination of docetaxel with cisplatin and fluorouracil. The combination of epirubicin, cisplatin, and fluorouracil (or capecitabine) is also commonly used.

48. What side effects can I expect from chemotherapy?

Depending on the chemotherapy treatments that you receive, you may experience multiple side effects, some side effects, or no side effects. After you and your doctor decide on your specific treatment, the doctor and nurse will discuss the possible side effects of treatment and the interventions to treat them. Each person responds to treatment differently, so you should not assume that you would necessarily have a side effect that another person has. Some possible side effects are the following:

- Nausea that may or may not be associated with vomiting. If this occurs, your physician may be able to prescribe antinausea medications. This will depend on your chemotherapy treatment and the severity of nausea. You may also be given intravenous fluid replacement, as some nausea can be attributed to dehydration.
- Vomiting can also be treated with antinausea medications. If the vomiting persists with the use of these medications, it is essential that you notify your physician to prevent dehydration. Intravenous fluid replacement is necessary at this point, as is medical intervention.
- Diarrhea can occur with certain treatments. It should always be controlled as soon as it is detected because it can also lead to dehydration. It is controlled with a BRAT diet (which consists of bananas, white rice, apple sauce, and white toast). It is also controlled with medications. If uncontrolled by diet and medication, your physician will physically assess you to make sure you don't have an infection and give you intravenous fluid replacement to alleviate dehydration.
- Constipation can occur as a direct result of antinausea medications, and may resolve on its own or with the help of mild laxatives or stool softeners. If constipation occurs for longer than 2 or 3 days, discuss this with your physician and nurse to assess for any additional problems and to assist with methods to alleviate the constipation.

Mucositis
Mouth sores
that may occur
with certain
chemotherapy
treatments.

Alopecia
Hair loss.

- **Mucositis,** or mouth sores, may also occur with certain chemotherapy treatments. This involves irritation to the lining of the mouth, back of the throat, and sometimes the tongue and lips. This can sometimes be prevented, but with certain treatments it is inevitable. There are over-the-counter (OTC) and prescription mouth treatments to treat mucositis. If you experience mucositis, you will have to change your diet until your symptoms subside. You should abstain from eating spicy foods, acidic foods, and any other foods that can irritate your mouth.

- **Alopecia,** or hair loss, is inevitable with certain chemotherapy agents. If you are receiving one of these treatments, you may want to consider cutting your hair short so that when hair loss begins, it may be less upsetting for you. You can invest in wigs, hair pieces, hats, and scarves as your tastes warrant. It is also important to realize that your hair loss is not permanent.

- Loss of fertility may be experienced by both male and female patients with the initiation of chemotherapy treatments. Women can begin to have irregular menstrual cycles and, in most cases, cease to menstruate as chemotherapy continues. If you are still within childbearing years or are interested in parenting your own children following treatment, it is important to discuss this with your health care team prior to starting treatment. Steps can be taken to bank sperm or harvest eggs for later use. It is essential to investigate these options prior to starting chemotherapy because eggs and sperm can be adversely affected by chemotherapy agents once treatments begin.

- Poor appetite can occur as a result of the disease or from chemotherapy treatment. Even if you do not feel like eating, it is essential to eat 5 to 6 small nutritious meals and snacks throughout the day. These can include foods that are high in protein, such as scrambled eggs, peanut butter, and cheese. It is easier for patients with stomach cancer to tolerate small meals. If you have a poor appetite, it is easier to eat a variety of smaller meals rather than 1 or 2 large meals that may be harder to consume.

- Fatigue can be attributed to your disease, treatment, or mental well-being. It is important that you allow yourself to rest when tired; eat small, frequent, well-balanced meals; and seek out the assistance of family and friends to help you with tasks and activities that you are unable to do by yourself. You should conserve your energy for those things that are the most important to you.

Activities that give you pleasure and make you feel good about yourself are what you want to save your energy for. Plan activities for the times during the day when your energy level is greater. If necessary, seek out your health care team if the fatigue persists, because you may need medical or psychosocial intervention. Fatigue can be the result of anemia or low red blood cell count. Medication is available to stimulate your bone marrow to make more red blood cells, which will raise your blood cell count and give you more energy.

Plan activities for the times during the day when your energy level is greater. If necessary, seek out your health care team if the fatigue persists, because you may need medical or psychosocial intervention. Fatigue can be the result of anemia or low red blood cell count.

If any of these side effects becomes prolonged or does not resolve with intervention, discuss the effects with your health care team.

Jim's comment:

I had most all of them at one time or another except for hair loss. My hair texture did change, especially after the radiation, but when everything was over the texture came back.

Ann's comment:

I think it's important to be a well-informed patient, but when it comes to learning about side effects, I'm of two minds. The drug companies have to tell you about every possible thing that can go wrong as a result of the drugs you're taking, but reading over that list can be a terrifying experience. On the other hand, no one would want to take a drug to cure one disease, only to have it cause another one. Except for losing my hair—that was shocking, but expected—the side effects of my chemo were minimal, with one exception. I was being followed for borderline glaucoma before I found out I had cancer. As a result of the steroids that were administered with the chemo, my optic pressures shot up into a dangerous range. Luckily, I had scheduled a routine appointment with my ophthalmologist during the chemo. He caught the problem right away and put me on medication to lower the pressures. Other than that, I had only minor problems until the last 2 ½ weeks, when I was getting chemo in conjunction with radiation. It was only then that I experienced low red and white blood counts, fatigue, and difficulty eating. The strangest side effect I had was a heightened sensitivity to ordinary smells like that of autumn leaves and pine boughs. (I had my chemotherapy in the fall and winter.) These and other smells, including some of my favorite restaurant aromas, made me feel queasy, and that sensation lasted for months after the end of chemo.

49. What major side effects will I experience with Cisplatin therapy?

The major side effects of Cisplatin can include numbness or tingling of the hands or feet, kidney damage, hair loss, nausea/vomiting, lowering of the blood counts, weakness, and fatigue.

Numbness or tingling usually starts slowly and worsens with continued treatment. If this becomes a serious problem, treatment will be stopped. Once treatment is stopped, this side effect slowly gets better but may not go away. Nausea and vomiting can usually be well controlled with antinausea medication. Hair loss, from very mild to almost complete, is common and reversible. Fatigue and weakness may be cumulative with treatment.

Rare but serious side effects with Cisplatin therapy include kidney damage, ringing in the ears, allergic reactions, blindness, heart attack, stroke, or seizures. These are usually associated with higher doses of Cisplatin therapy.

The side effects of Cisplatin can be minimized with reduced drug dosing. So, for this reason, often Cisplatin is given at a lower dose weekly instead of a large dose every 4 weeks.

50. What are the major side effects of docetaxel therapy?

Potential side effects of docetaxel therapy include fatigue, diarrhea, and hair loss. Side effects may also include mouth sores, headaches, muscle and joint aches, swelling in the ankles, rash, nail discoloration, drop in the blood counts (which may result in infection), and drop in blood-clotting platelets (which may result in easy bruising).

Rare but serious side effects may include damage to small nerves in the body, resulting in numbness or tingling in the fingers and toes. This may be long lasting and occurs in a minority of patients. If you experience numbness or tingling in your fingers or toes, the dose of docetaxel may be reduced. Docetaxel may cause an allergic reaction. You will be asked to take dexamethasone (Decadron®, Merck) 4 to 8 mg the evening before, the morning of, and the evening after each dose of docetaxel to decrease your risk of allergic reaction and minimize side effects from docetaxel.

51. What are potential side effects with fluorouracil therapy?

It is likely that you will experience a drop in blood counts, including white blood cells. Diarrhea, nausea, vomiting, loss of appetite, fatigue, abdominal pain or cramps, mouth sores or sores in the throat or esophagus, nail changes, and skin darkening are also common. Less likely side effects may include watery eyes, eye irritation, blurred vision, nose stuffiness, hives, itching, headaches, shortness of breath, and blistering of the palms of the hands and soles of the feet.

Rare, but serious, effects may include unsteadiness of movement, severe life-threatening diarrhea, heart attack or chest pain, and blood clots.

52. What are the common chemotherapy side effects with irinotecan?

The major side effects of irinotecan may include diarrhea, lowering of the blood counts, and fatigue. Diarrhea may occur during or immediately after irinotecan, or after a few days of treatment. Early diarrhea may be associated with abdominal cramping and is readily treatable with antidiarrheal medication. Late diarrhea is treated immediately with Imodium. However, if severe diarrhea occurs, you may need to be admitted to the hospital for intravenous fluids.

Irinotecan can lower your blood counts. The white cells (infection fighting) are most susceptible. This may temporarily put you at risk for an infection. Should you develop a fever (101.5°F or greater, or if you don't feel right), you may have a potentially life-threatening infection and must notify your doctor immediately. You may need to be admitted to the hospital for intravenous antibiotics until your blood count is at a safe level. Diarrhea that occurs when the white blood cells are low is worrisome, as death has resulted from this combination of side effects. The risk of this happening is low, but do inform your doctor of any side effect you may be experiencing.

Irinotecan, at higher doses, may cause mouth sores. If this happens, you will be given a mouthwash that soothes the mouth and gums. Irinotecan is also associated with the development of blood clots, particularly in combination with other chemotherapy, including cisplatin.

53. What are standard chemotherapy options for stomach cancer?

As previously discussed, several chemotherapy drugs are active in the treatment of advanced or metastatic stomach and GEJ cancer. Because there are several options, to some extent the treatments can be tailored to the individual patient. For example, irinotecan is a drug that is known to cause diarrhea. If a patient has underlying inflammatory bowel disease (such as Crohn's disease or ulcerative colitis), he or she would be more prone to having diarrhea. In this case, the patient would opt to avoid irinotecan as part of a treatment plan. Another example is the use of cisplatin in older patients who may have some renal impairment. Cisplatin is cleared by the kidneys, and in the setting of even modest kidney impairment, it can damage the kidneys even further and may be associated with even more side effects. So, in these patients, cisplatin would be avoided.

Generally, most drugs have modest activity against the cancer and can be given without major side effects. Because different chemotherapy classes are active, the drugs can be combined to increase the antitumor effects against the cancer. However, with each combination, you run the risk of increasing side effects. These are discussed in more detail next.

Several combination therapies have been tested and are commonly used. For most patients, cisplatin and fluorouracil-based treatment will be the most appropriate. Some important combinations to know about include the following:

- Cisplatin + Fluorouracil
  In this combination, cisplatin is given on the first day (or sometimes the first and second day), and fluorouracil is given as a continuous infusion over 4 to 5 days. This combination has been tested the most, historically, but is not as commonly used because of side effects, which include nausea, vomiting, weakness, mouth sores, diarrhea, and a drop in the blood counts.

Generally, most drugs have modest activity against the cancer and can be given without major side effects. Because different chemotherapy classes are active, the drugs can be combined to increase the antitumor effects against the cancer.

- Docetaxel + Cisplatin + Fluorouracil (or Docetaxel + Cisplatin)
  This combination is similar to cisplatin + fluorouracil (described above) but with the addition of docetaxel. This was examined in the TAX325 study and was proven to be superior to cisplatin + fluorouracil, with about equal gastrointestinal side effects. Because of the side effects of this regimen, selecting the right patient to receive it is important. Currently, active areas of research involve finding better ways to combine these three drugs to make them easier to take. It is common to use the same combination without fluorouracil, for example, docetaxel + cisplatin. Without fluorouracil, the side effects of mouth sores and diarrhea are lessened.
- Epirubicin + Cisplatin + Fluorouracil
  This combination was developed originally in England. Here, the fluorouracil is given as a continuous infusion for 21 straight days. Because patients are constantly physically tied to the fluorouracil infusion pump, they may not prefer this option. However, it does have very good activity in the treatment of stomach and GEJ cancers, and it also works for localized disease (see Question 39). More recently, clinical studies showed that the continuous infusion of fluorouracil may be substituted by an oral form of fluorouracil called capecitabine. This change makes the regimen much more convenient.
- Irinotecan + Cisplatin
  This combination is active in the treatment of stomach and GEJ cancer but is less commonly used. In Japan and Europe, cisplatin is given at a high dose every 3 or 4 weeks, and irinotecan is given weekly. When given this way, side effects are greater and may interfere with the benefit of the regimen. In the United States, the most common way the combination is given is together weekly for 2 weeks in a row, followed by a 1-week break.

- Oxaliplatin + Fluorouracil/Leucovorin (FOLFOX)
  This regimen is also very active in the treatment of
  stomach cancer. Recent studies have demonstrated that
  oxaliplatin can be substituted for cisplatin in the treatment of advanced disease. Oxaliplatin is less toxic to
  the kidneys and is more tolerable in many ways, making
  this regimen very attractive. Also, very interestingly, this
  regimen works after trying cisplatin-based treatments,
  suggesting that the regimen indeed is quite active.

54. What are the common side effects of combination Epirubicin/Cisplatin/5FU (ECF) therapy?

The most common side effects of (ECF) Epirubicin/Cisplatin/
5FU are the following:

- Patients can have pink-tinged urine for 24 to 48 hours
  post-infusion because the medication is pink.
- Mouth sores are very common because both epirubicin
  and 5FU (fluouracil) cause this side effect.
- Fatigue is quite common during the first week of treatment when all three drugs are given, but it resolves as
  the week progresses. In weeks 2 and 3 of treatment,
  when you get only 5FU, your energy level usually nor-
  malizes. As you are exposed to more and more chemotherapy, the fatigue can increase, as most side effects are
  cumulative.
- Skin discoloration and darkening is a common side
  effect of 5FU and epirubicin. Both pick up on the
  pigment that is already in your skin and can cause the
  color of your nail beds to deepen. The color of the skin
  on your hands and feet may darken, especially if you
  already have a dark complexion. If you are prone to
  brown spots, they may deepen in color, or more of them
  may develop.

- Diarrhea is common with infusional 5FU. The diarrhea can usually be controlled when treated immediately.
- **Myelosuppression** is common with most chemotherapy drugs and regimens. With ECF therapy, it is usual for this to happen: a drop in the levels of the white blood cells, which are the infection-fighting cells of your body (e.g., WBC and absolute neutrophil count, ANC), and platelets.
- Delayed nausea and vomiting are common following cisplatin and epirubicin therapy. To offset this problem, medications are given for two days following the infusion of these two drugs.
- It is possible for kidney damage to occur if the patient doesn't drink enough after cisplatin therapy. Patients should drink 1.5 to 2 liters of fluid daily after getting cisplatin.
- Mild neuropathic (nerve) pain can occur in the hands and feet as a result of exposure to cisplatin.
- Watery eyes and a runny nose occur as a result of the continuous infusion of 5FU.
- Hair loss can occur but is not a certainty.

Myelosuppression

A condition in which bone marrow activity is decreased, resulting in fewer red blood cells, white blood cells, and platelets. Myelosuppression is a side effect of some cancer treatments.

55. What are the common side effects of Docetaxel/Cisplatin/Fluorouracil (DCF) therapy?

- Myelosuppression is common with most chemotherapy drugs and regimens. With DCF therapy, it is usual to see a drop in the white blood counts and the platelets.
- Hair loss will occur, usually following the second or third treatment.
- Neuropathic (nerve) pain can occur in the hands and feet as a result of exposure to cisplatin and docetaxel. It usually occurs after 3 to 4 treatments.
- Delayed nausea and vomiting may occur following cisplatin. Medications are given to offset this problem for two days following the infusion of this drug.

- Kidney damage can occur if you do not drink enough, and particularly if you are unable to drink because of nausea or if you become dehydrated due to diarrhea. Patients should drink 1.5 to 2 liters of fluid daily after getting cisplatin.
- Fatigue is quite common. As you are exposed to more and more chemotherapy, fatigue usually increases as the side effects are cumulative.
- Skin discoloration and darkening is a common side effect of 5FU therapy. The pigment that is already in your skin and nail beds deepens in color. The color of your hands and feet may darken, especially if you already have a dark complexion. If you are prone to brown spots, they may deepen in color, or more of them may develop.
- Changes in nail texture may occur. They may thicken, get ridges, and become brittle and peel as a result of the docetaxel.
- There is a possibility of mouth sores from the 5FU infusion. Medications such as Gelclair® (EKR Therapeutics) can help reduce the severity of mouth sores.
- There is a small possibility of diarrhea from the 5FU infusion. This is usually controlled with medications.
- Watery eyes and a runny nose may occur as a result of 5FU or docetaxel.

56. What are the most common side effects of Irinotecan (CPT-11)/Cisplatin therapy?

- Diarrhea can occur after the first treatment, but more commonly after 2 to 3 cycles (6 to 9 weeks).
- Hair loss can occur after 1 or 2 cycles (up to 3 to 6 weeks).
- Mild neuropathic (nerve) pain can occur in the hands and feet as a result of exposure to cisplatin.
- Myelosuppression is common with most chemotherapy drugs and regimens. A drop in the WBC, ANC, and platelet counts can be expected.

Treatment Options

- Delayed nausea and vomiting may occur after receiving cisplatin, but for two days following infusion of it, medications can be given to offset this problem.
- It is possible for kidney damage to occur if the patient does not hydrate well enough after receiving cisplatin. Patients should drink 1.5 to 2 liters of fluid daily after getting cisplatin.
- Fatigue is common, and the more chemotherapy you are exposed to, the more fatigue you will have.

57. What are the most common side effects of FOLFOX (5fu/leucovorin/ oxaliplatin) therapy?

- Myelosuppression is common with most chemotherapy drugs and regimens. A drop in the WBC, ANC, and platelet counts can be expected.
- Neuropathic (nerve) pain can occur in the hands and feet as a result of exposure to oxaliplatin.
- There is a small possibility of mouth sores from the infusion of 5FU.
- There is a possibility of diarrhea from the 5FU infusion, which is usually controlled with medications.
- You can have severe throat pain when swallowing cold beverages for 2 to 3 days post-oxaliplatin therapy.
- You can have cold sensitivity in your fingertips when touching cold substances 2 to 3 days post-oxaliplatin therapy
- Nausea and vomiting may occur and can be controlled with medications.
- Fatigue is a common complaint. The more chemotherapy you are exposed to, the more fatigue you will have, as the side effects are cumulative.
- Skin discoloration and darkening are common with 5FU. The nail beds may deepen in color. The color of your hands and feet may darken, especially if you already have a dark complexion. If you are prone to brown spots, they may deepen in color, or more of them may develop.

- Watery eyes and a runny nose may occur as a result of 5FU.
- Hair loss may occur

58. Can I use herbal or botanical products along with the therapy my doctor recommends?

The use of herbal medications and botanical products is something that you must always discuss with your oncologist and health care team. It is essential to stop using any botanical products until they are properly approved by your doctor. Many familiar botanical products can cause adverse problems when used in conjunction with chemotherapy treatments and other commonly used medications. In many cases, botanical products interfere with the metabolism of prescribed medications, causing an increased or decreased amount of the medication in your system. This can lead to drug toxicity or decreased effectiveness. Some botanical products may exacerbate the side effects of cancer therapy drugs.

Most large cancer care centers have an integrative medicine department that incorporates natural, holistic treatment methodologies with more common, modern medical cancer treatments in a safe and reliable setting. If your treatment center does not have an integrative medicine department, discuss any possible botanical treatments with your health care team prior to taking them.

Most large cancer care centers have an integrative medicine department that incorporates natural, holistic treatment methodologies with more common, modern medical cancer treatments in a safe and reliable setting.

59. What is a Mediport or portacath, and what are they used for?

Mediports and **portocaths** are devices that access a central vein used for giving chemotherapy. In a minor surgical procedure by a surgeon or radiologist, they are generally placed under the skin pocket in the upper chest wall or upper arm.

In gastric and GEJ cancers, the devices are used mainly for giving chemotherapy over days continuously, most commonly

Mediports/ portocaths
Devices that access a central vein used for giving chemotherapy.

fluorouracil. Fluorouracil can be prepared by a pharmacist in a portable pump that can be attached to the port so that the treatment can be administered continuously.

During the first few days after receiving the port, a patient should try to avoid heavy exertion. It is also important to access the port under sterile conditions, as these internal devices are prone to infection.

60. What new drugs are on the horizon, and how can I find out about them?

Over the past 5 years, there has been an explosion of new research done to understand how cancer cells work. By better understanding the way cancer cells operate, we hope to identify specific areas of vulnerability that we can exploit with **designer drugs**, also called *targeted* or *biologic drugs*. There has been recent success with this approach in many cancers. For example, bevacizumab (Avastin®, Genentech Inc.) is a new targeted drug that is an antibody against a normal protein called Vascular Endothelial Growth Factor, or VEGF. This protein stimulates new blood vessels to grow. By binding to this protein, bevacizumab blocks its function on the endothelial cells of blood vessels, thereby stunting its growth. Bevacizumab is perhaps the first drug in a growing new class of anticancer drugs called **anti-angiogenesis agents**—drugs that attack the blood vessels to tumors. Most excitingly, the combination of chemotherapy with bevacizumab has proven to be beneficial in many malignancies, including colorectal cancer, breast cancer, and lung cancer. The addition of bevacizumab has been tested in stomach cancer, and early results show some promise for its use in stomach cancer. Research on this drug and other drugs like it is ongoing. Other anti-angiogenesis drugs that have shown recent promise include sorafanib (Nexavar®, Bayer Pharmaceuticals Inc.), sunitinib (Sutent®, Pfizer Inc.), and VEGF-Trap (Sanofi-Aventis, Inc.).

Designer drugs

Drugs developed specifically to attack the cancer at a very specific and critical target or pathway.

Anti-angiogenesis agents

Drugs that attack the blood vessels to tumors.

Another class of biologic drugs is the **Epidermal Growth Factor Receptor Inhibitors**, or **EGFR inhibitors**. Cetuximab (Erbitux®, Imclone Inc.) and panitumumab (Vectibix®, Amgen Pharmaceuticals Inc.) are antibodies that block the EGF receptor on cells. They have proven activity in colorectal cancer and head and neck cancer (cetuximab only), and are actively being tested in gastric and esophageal cancers.

These two new classes of anticancer drugs are just the tip of the iceberg. Over the next several decades, hundreds of other drugs that are directed at new targets within the cancer cell will be tested. Several of them will show benefit. The process of testing new drugs and treatments for cancer is conducted by clinical trials. These trials often offer patients an opportunity to have access to new drugs that are not yet approved for use by the FDA (see Question 61). The NCI Web site and your physician can also guide you toward these new and evolving treatment options.

61. What is a clinical trial?

A **clinical trial** is a research study designed to test a specific treatment on humans. This treatment may be a new drug, a new combination of drugs, radiation therapy, biologics, or a new drug for a different disease. Clinical trials may also involve nutritional and behavioral therapies. Most new treatments are developed in the laboratory and then tested in animals. If it is deemed safe in animals, it is then tested in the human population for safety and effectiveness. There are three phases of clinical trials.

- The first phase is done to determine the appropriate dose, frequency, and side effects of the medication or regimen. In this phase, safety is of primary concern. These studies include a limited number of patients who would not be helped by standard treatments.
- The second phase determines the efficacy of the treatment regimen. These trials also test for new treatments

Epidermal Growth Factor Receptor Inhibitors

A class of biologic drugs that block the signaling from a cellular receptor called the epidermal growth factor receptor.

Clinical trial

A research study designed to test a specific treatment on humans. This treatment may be a new drug, a new combination of drugs, radiation therapy, biologics, or a new drug for a different disease.

Most new treatments are developed in the laboratory and then tested in animals. If it is deemed safe in animals, it is then tested in the human population for safety and effectiveness.

Treatment Options

against a specific cancer. These trials involve small numbers of patients and have unknown risks associated with them.

- The third phase, or Phase 3, trials are done to determine efficacy as compared to the current standard of care for that particular disease. These trials often include large numbers of patients and are conducted nationwide. Patients in this type of study are randomly assigned to one of two groups in which one group will receive the standard regimen and the other will receive the new regimen. They do not have a choice as to which group they are assigned.

Strict guidelines must be followed when on a clinical trial. The Food and Drug Administration (FDA) regulates how these trials are conducted. The study is also approved by an Investigational Review Board (IRB) at the hospital where the trial originates. Each trial has specific eligibility criteria. Patients must sign a consent form that describes the study, side effects, financial obligations, and risks and benefits of the trial.

There are benefits of participating in a clinical trial: receiving new treatments before they are commercially available, constant monitoring, and access to academic cancer institutions.

There are benefits of participating in a clinical trial: receiving new treatments before they are commercially available, constant monitoring, and access to academic cancer institutions. It is important to remember, though, that the treatment given in clinical trials has not been proven to be superior to the current standard of care. Patients may experience more side effects and extra financial costs, and they may receive additional diagnostic tests.

Ann's comment:

I was considered for a clinical trial at the cancer center where I was treated. I even signed a consent form and was given a thick document outlining the protocol. Reading that document was probably a mistake, because at the time, I was very new to the world of cancer and cancer research. When I got to the part about possible side effects of the drugs that would be administered, it was so frighten-

ing, I burst into tears. I decided I didn't want to participate. But after speaking to a colleague who was very knowledgeable about cancer, I changed my mind and tried to get into the trial. In the end, I was deemed ineligible. But if I were in that situation again, I'm pretty sure I'd jump at the chance to participate. Having been through one cancer ordeal, I think it would be a little easier not to worry about all the things that could go wrong in a trial.

62. How do I find out about a clinical trial that is appropriate for me?

Most patients get involved in a clinical trial by invitation from their current physician.

You should consult with your physician to determine whether a clinical trial is right for you and if so, which ongoing trials may be appropriate for you. Or, you can call 800-4-CANCER (National Institutes of Health) to get a list of clinical trials. You can also contact the National Comprehensive Cancer Network (NCCN) at *www.nccn.org* to find out whether there are any available trials that are appropriate for you.

Jim's comment:

I was in a clinical trial, and while I have no other experience, I believe I got the best and most advanced treatment available.

63. How important are statistics for each individual patient?

Survival statistics cannot predict a prognosis for a particular individual, but instead measure the 5-year survival of all patients with a similar diagnosis. The **5-year survival rate** means the percentage of patients who live for at least 5 years after they are diagnosed with cancer. These rates are used as a standard way of discussing prognosis. Survival depends on numerous characteristics, such as your overall health, response to treatment, and stage of disease.

5-year survival rate

The percentage of patients who live for at least 5 years after they are diagnosed with cancer.

The overall 5-year survival rate of all people with stomach cancer in the United States is about 20% to 25%. This survival rate has improved only slightly in the last 15 years. One reason for this is that most stomach cancers in the United States are diagnosed at an advanced rather than early stage. The stage of the cancer is very important in determining the prognosis (outlook for survival) for patients. Another factor is the location of the cancer. The 5-year survival rate for cancers of the proximal stomach (the upper portion of the stomach closest to the esophagus) is lower than for cancers in the distal stomach (the lower portion of the stomach closest to the small intestine).

It is important to remember that statistics on cancer survival are only averages. You cannot predict your survival outlook based on these statistics.

It is important to remember that statistics on cancer survival are only averages. You cannot predict your survival outlook based on these statistics. Many people survive longer than would be expected based on their stage of cancer.

Ann's comment:

I just about lost it when I heard the survival statistics for stomach cancer. Luckily, I have an optimistic husband who insisted on seeing me as a survivor, and I had a compassionate surgeon who helped me get some perspective on the statistics. Among other things, the surgeon referred me to an essay titled "The Median Isn't the Message" by the evolutionary biologist Stephen Jay Gould. It's easy to find on the Internet, and it offers some hope to those who have been diagnosed with an aggressive form of cancer. Even now, I find the survival statistics alarming, but the shock of hearing them for the first time—like so many other aspects of the disease—diminished over time. My surgeon once suggested that I adopt the approach of another of his patients: She put her cancer experience—the diagnosis, treatment, survival statistics, and so forth—into a box, shut the lid, and only opened it up when she saw her doctors for checkups. I don't think I'm as skillful as she is at "compartmentalizing," but it's something to work toward.

64. Will my insurance plan cover my cancer treatments?

When you and your physicians decide what your treatment will include and at what health care facility you will be receiving treatment, you should contact your insurance carrier. Most insurance carriers have a patient contact telephone line that allows you to discuss what each plan will cover. A patient may want to have a close family member or friend manage these insurance issues, as it can be extremely stressful to worry about financial concerns when trying to handle a new cancer diagnosis.

It is important to know whether your plan will cover not only the cost of the actual treatments but also physician visits, blood work, diagnostic examinations (including CT scans, x-rays, pet scans, and so forth), and, most importantly, the at-home medications that you may need for chemotherapy side effects.

Some insurance plans cover the majority of treatments but specify that certain diagnostic testing and medications need prior authorization or approval from the doctor's office. You may also need approval before starting treatment from the medical management department of your insurance company.

It is essential to have this information in advance to avoid any unnecessary bills and stress that these financial pressures add during this already stressful time.

Some insurance plans cover the majority of treatments but specify that certain diagnostic testing and medications need prior authorization or approval from the doctor's office.

65. How does my doctor know whether my treatment is working? What if my treatment doesn't work?

Prior to starting chemotherapy, your doctor will try to get a good assessment of how advanced the disease is and where it is located. Generally, a CT (computer-assisted tomography) scan is used to get this assessment. The CT scan does a good job of viewing any spots that might be in the abdomen, lymph nodes, or lungs. Often, intravenous contrast and oral contrast are required to see cancer deposits in the liver or within the abdomen itself.

After we have a good baseline evaluation, chemotherapy is given for a period of two to three months. Following treatment, a repeat CT scan is performed, and the two scans (baseline scan and the current scan) are compared to one another. The nature of cancer is to grow. If the CT scan shows that the stomach cancer has not grown or has decreased in size, this means that the chemotherapy treatment is controlling the disease and stopping the cancer from growing. If there is no sign that the cancer has progressed or metastasized and you are tolerating your treatment, the doctor will continue the treatment regimen for as long as it is controlling the cancer. The treatment may be given for a specific number of cycles or indefinitely. However, if the CT scan shows that the cancer has grown or metastasized, this would suggest that the current treatment is not working and alternative treatments should be sought.

The doctor will also perform routine physical exams, blood tests, and radiologic studies to check the status of your cancer. The types of blood tests and radiologic studies will depend on the stage and type of stomach cancer that you have.

Throughout your course of treatment, you will be visiting your doctor regularly. During these visits, he or she will evaluate you to see how you are doing. The visits are important to determine how well you are tolerating treatment, what side effects (if any) you may be experiencing, and the severity of those side effects. Depending on the side effects, your doctor may order medication to help relieve them, or adjust the dose or schedule of your treatment regimen.

Throughout your course of treatment, you will be visiting your doctor regularly. During these visits, he or she will evaluate you to see how you are doing. The visits are important to determine how well you are tolerating treatment, what side effects (if any) you may be experiencing, and the severity of those side effects.

Getting clear and accurate information from your doctor is very important. This will allow you to make knowledgeable decisions about what comes next. If you were hoping for a cure, hearing that your disease has progressed may make you rethink your treatment goals. You may want to communicate these goals to your physician, significant other, and other family members. Being knowledgeable about your treatment options and plan of care is a good way to help you make the best decision about your care. A resource that may be useful during this time is *When Cancer Recurs: Meeting the Challenge*, published by the National Cancer Institute.

66. Is a CT (CAT) scan always helpful?

CT scans are not always helpful. Most of the time, a CT scan will show the sites of disease that are outside of the stomach or abdomen. However, about a third of the time, cancer of the stomach spreads only to the abdomen or on the surface of the intestines, called the peritoneum. In this situation, the CT scan may not clearly see the disease that is within the wall of the stomach or of the intestines. Additionally, stomach cancer by nature can grow sideways within the stomach or intestinal wall. In this event, you may have symptoms of abdominal cramping, nausea, and/or loss of appetite caused by the disease within the wall that impairs the function of the stomach and intestines. Importantly, when the cancer grows within the intestinal wall, it is not easily identifiable on the CT scan or on other types of scans; the tumor mass often cannot be seen on cross-sectional imaging, so the CT scan may not show the disease at all. This can sometimes make treatment decisions difficult. Patients may be asked about their bowel function and, more specifically, whether they have noticed any weight loss. Patients will also be asked about their eating habits and whether they are able to eat enough to maintain their weight. They may notice some abdominal cramps or increased weakness. If these symptoms existed prior to starting therapy and have since improved, this would indicate that the treatment was working. However, if these symptoms seem to be worsening, this may suggest either that the chemotherapy is too strong and these are side effects or that the treatment is not working. In either case, an adjustment should be made: either lower the dose or give additional medications to alleviate chemotherapy side effects, or else switch to alternative chemotherapeutic agents.

67. What other scans are useful in stomach cancer?

There are other radiographic studies that may be useful to monitor your disease beyond the use of a CT scan. Some patients may have an allergy to intravenous contrast that is used for CT scans. The contrast used for CT scans typically involves the use of an iodine-based material. Some people have an allergy to iodine and are unable to receive the intravenous contrast or may only be able to receive it if they are premedicated with steroids. The intravenous contrast is used to identify lesions in the liver and abdomen. An alternative imaging study that is sometimes used is magnetic resonance imaging, known as an MRI with gadolinium contrast. Most patients are not allergic to gadolinium and can receive this intravenous contrast agent for use in MRI testing without difficulty.

Currently, the PET scan is most commonly used to identify sites of disease within your body that were not well seen on the CT scan.

A newer test to monitor your disease is called a PET scan (positron emission tomography). In this scan, a small amount of sugar is tagged with radiation. This sugar is taken up by metabolically active cells within the body. For example, your heart or brain is metabolically active and will take up this radioactive sugar. The areas that take up this radioactive sugar will light up as positive on the PET scan; these are normal structures that should light up. Your cancer is also metabolically active and will light up with uptake of this radioactive sugar in about two-thirds of cases. Currently, the PET scan is most commonly used to identify sites of disease within your body that were not well seen on the CT scan. Current research is ongoing to investigate the use of PET scans to monitor the response of the cancer to chemotherapy.

68. What is palliative care?

Palliative care is a term that encompasses medical, physical, emotional, spiritual, and social well-being. It is care that is directed to helping patients achieve the best quality of life possible. It is given with the intent to prolong survival and improve symptoms, but not as a cure. Palliative care no longer refers to just hospice care, but now includes any patient who may benefit from this approach to treatment. Patients who are currently receiving treatment and have a good prognosis may also benefit from palliative care.

Palliative care specialists, physicians trained to manage pain and other symptoms, may be consulted. If your pain or other symptoms are not well managed, you should ask your doctor about seeing a palliative care specialist.

Palliative care

Care that is not curative and encompasses medical, physical, emotional, spiritual, and social well-being. It is directed at helping patients achieve the best quality of life.

69. What palliative treatments are available to treat gastric cancer?

For metastatic gastric cancer, chemotherapy is considered palliative. This means that it is given to improve survival and quality of life. Other palliative therapies include the following:

- Endoscopic laser surgery or endoluminal stent placement as palliative therapy to relieve symptoms and improve the quality of life
- Radiation therapy as palliative therapy to stop bleeding, relieve pain, or shrink a tumor that is blocking the opening to the stomach
- Surgery as palliative therapy to stop bleeding or shrink a tumor that is blocking the opening to the stomach
- A catheter, such as a Tenckhoff® catheter, can be placed into the abdomen to drain troublesome fluid, called ascites, that can develop in that cavity from the cancer. By draining this fluid, symptoms of bloating or breathing problems may improve.

For metastatic gastric cancer, chemotherapy is considered palliative. This means that it is given to improve survival and quality of life.

70. Will I have pain? What are my choices if I experience pain?

Not everyone who has cancer will experience pain. You may experience pain based on the location of your tumor. If a tumor grows or spreads and presses on a nerve or invades a surrounding organ, you may experience pain. Procedures used to diagnose and treat cancer may also cause pain. Pain has always been considered a normal part of having cancer. With the development of new pain medications and greater knowledge of how to use these pain medications to effectively treat pain, it can be well controlled in most people.

There is no benefit to having pain. Many people are worried or concerned about taking pain medications. Pain is not a part of cancer that you have to accept, nor will taking pain medication mask a problem or diminish response to treatment. Having pain can be disabling, regardless of severity. Pain can affect your appetite, ability to sleep, mood, and energy level. You should tell your doctor about any discomfort or pain that you are experiencing. Pain can vary from one person to another, and it can manifest as discomfort, aching, cramping, or a sharp stabbing sensation. Describing your pain accurately to your nurse or physician will help them prescribe a medication that is appropriate for you. In describing your pain, include the location of pain, severity of pain (0 to 10 scale, with 0 being no pain and 10 being the worst imaginable pain), duration of pain (chronic or only at certain times during the day), what increases or relieves your pain, and how it affects your quality of life.

Analgesics are medications that treat pain. Analgesics vary in strength and are usually given in a stepwise fashion. Mild analgesics may be given first and increased to a stronger analgesic until your pain is well controlled. Over-the-counter (OTC) analgesics such as acetaminophen, aspirin, and ibuprofen are considered first-line analgesics and are available

---

Pain is not a part of cancer that you have to accept, nor will taking pain medication mask a problem or diminish response to treatment. Having pain can be disabling, regardless of severity. Pain can affect your appetite, ability to sleep, mood, and energy level. You should tell your doctor about any discomfort or pain that you are experiencing.

Analgesics

Medications that treat pain.

without a prescription. Nonsteroidal anti-inflammatory drugs (NSAIDs) such as COX-2 inhibitors (celecoxib, rofecoxib, valdecoxib) are less irritating to the stomach but require a prescription. If your pain is not controlled by one of these medications, your doctor will prescribe an opioid or narcotic analgesic (morphine, hydromorphone, oxycodone, fentanyl). Other medications are also effective when used with analgesics to treat pain, including some antidepressants, anticonvulsants, and steroids.

Medications for pain come in a variety of dosage forms. These can be tablets, capsules, liquids (swallowed or taken sublingually), skin patches, and rectal suppositories. Pain medication can also be given intravenously (into the vein via a pump). These portable pumps can be set to deliver a constant dose of medication with "extra" doses as needed. This type of pump is called a **PCA pump**, or patient controlled analgesia pump, whereby the patient determines when he or she needs some extra pain relief.

PCA pump

Patient controlled analgesic pump, whereby the patient determines when he or she needs some extra pain relief.

Chronic pain is effectively treated when pain medication is given continuously or around the clock. This allows for a steady or constant level of pain medication in your blood to prevent you from experiencing pain. Pain can be controlled by taking long-acting pain medications because they have a long duration of action, meaning that their effect can last from many hours to days. To help control breakthrough or intermittent pain, an immediate-release medication can be given. These medications work quickly and are short-acting. Breakthrough pain is pain or discomfort experienced while you are on long-acting medication. If you wait too long between doses of long-acting medication and your pain worsens, the medication will not work as quickly or effectively. If you find you are using your immediate-release medication frequently or are experiencing a lot of pain, you should talk to your doctor about increasing your dose of long-acting pain medication.

Pain varies from person to person, so what works for you may not work as well for someone else. It may take some time to find the right pain medication, dose, and frequency to control your pain. Work with your doctor and nurse until you find a regimen that works for you. If you are still not satisfied with the level of pain relief that you are experiencing, ask them about a referral to a pain specialist.

71. What follow-up do I need after my treatment?

Follow-up care after treatment for stomach cancer is important. Even when there are no longer any signs of cancer, the disease sometimes returns because undetected cancer cells remained somewhere in the body after treatment. Your doctor will monitor your recovery and check for recurrence of the cancer. Checkups help ensure that any changes in your health are noted and treated if needed. Checkups will include a physical exam, lab tests, and periodic x-rays, CT scans, endoscopies, or other tests. Between scheduled visits, you should contact the doctor if you have any health problems.

Your doctor will monitor your recovery and check for recurrence of the cancer. Checkups help ensure that any changes in your health are noted and treated if needed.

72. What is the distinction between home care and home health care?

Home care, also known as domiciliary care, is health care provided in the patient's home by either health care professionals or by family and friends. Often, though, the term *home care* is used to distinguish nonmedical or custodial care from care provided by licensed professionals. In this sense, home care is care that is provided by people who are not nurses, doctors, or other licensed medical personnel. The term **home health care** refers to care that is provided by licensed and trained medical personnel.

Home care

Health care provided in the patient's home by either health care professionals or by family and friends.

Home health care

Care provided by licensed and trained medical personnel.

Some cancer patients have the option to receive care at home so that they can feel more comfortable and secure. Many patients want to stay at home so that they will not be separated from family, friends, and familiar surroundings. Home care can help patients achieve this desire. It often involves a team approach that includes doctors, nurses, social workers, physical therapists, family members, and others.

Services provided by home care agencies may include access to medical equipment; visits from registered nurses, physical therapists, and social workers; help with running errands, meal preparation, and personal hygiene; and delivery of medication. The state or local health department is another important resource in finding home care services. Your local health department should have a registry of licensed home care agencies.

Treatment Options

PART SIX

Living with Gastric Cancer

Will I lose my hair with chemotherapy?

When am I cured of stomach cancer?

How can I cope with the fear of recurrence?

More . . .

73. Will I lose my hair with chemotherapy?

This depends on the specific chemotherapy agent that you will receive. When you and your health care provider discuss your chemotherapy regimen, you should ask about the possibility and/or likelihood of hair loss. Some chemotherapy agents cause hair thinning while others cause total hair loss. This hair loss is usually not permanent, and your hair does start to grow back between treatments, or when treatment ends or changes.

Some options for dealing with hair loss include wigs, head wraps, and hats. Also, cutting your hair very short may make the loss less traumatizing. It is important to know that some insurance plans cover wigs for chemotherapy-related hair loss.

Some options for dealing with hair loss include wigs, head wraps, and hats. Also, cutting your hair very short may make the loss less traumatizing. It is important to know that some insurance plans cover wigs for chemotherapy-related hair loss. You should check your specific plan to see if this is an option for you. Wigs can vary in price, from inexpensive to very expensive.

Jim's comment:

I never lost my hair, but it did change texture while I was undergoing my treatments.

Ann's comment:

I knew I would lose my hair after I began chemotherapy—I just didn't know when. For several weeks, nothing seemed to change, and I think I started to believe that it wasn't going to happen. Then one day, standing in front of the bathroom mirror, I was combing my hair and it just started coming out in clumps. It was very dramatic—and upsetting. Since I didn't want it to keep coming out in handfuls, I went to my husband's barber and had him give me a buzz cut. Eventually, I lost even the duck fuzz, but the baldness stopped bothering me pretty quickly. Weeks earlier, I'd gotten a wig for free at the cancer center where I was treated, but I never wore it. Whenever I went out, I wore a headscarf. When I went to the gym, I wore a baseball cap. I never once felt as though I stood out. Luckily, I live in a city where so many people have unusual or eccentric styles of dress that no one even seemed to notice my headgear.

74. Will I be able to have intercourse with my partner during treatments?

The answer to this depends a great deal on your particular situation: how recently you had surgery, your childbearing status, and your general physical and mental health.

If you have recently had surgery, you should wait until you get medical clearance from your surgeon before resuming sexual activity with your partner.

If you are receiving chemotherapy and either you or your partner is still within childbearing years, you *must* use double barrier contraception (this includes condoms and a form of female contraception). This is necessary to prevent pregnancy because the effects of chemotherapy on the egg, sperm, and fetus are unknown, and possibly very dangerous.

However, if you are physically able and mentally willing to participate in sexual activities with your partner, you should do so. It is important that people assume as much of a normal life as possible when on treatment. The take-home message should always be to assume the best quality of life as possible.

Jim's comment:

My wife and I were beyond the childbearing stage and we continued our normal sexual activities.

75. I am having problems getting or maintaining an erection since treatment. How can this be treated?

Erectile dysfunction is the inability to get and/or maintain an erection. Cancer and its treatment may affect erectile function. Sexual desire and energy level change during treatment, but

Erectile dysfunction

The inability to have and/or maintain an erection.

it is normal and can happen for a number of reasons. Erectile dysfunction may interfere with sexuality and physical intimacy. Good communication is an important part of sexual intimacy. A partner's concerns or fears are a normal part of the sexual relationship but can negatively impact the sexual experience if they are not openly communicated.

There are four phases of sexual response in men. The first phase is the desire for intimacy. The second phase is excitement. Blood vessels in the penis open up, and the increased blood flow in the penis causes it to become "hard." The third phase is orgasm. This is the sensation of pleasure and when ejaculation happens. The last phase is when blood drains out of the penis and the penis loses its erection.

Erectile dysfunction in men could be the result of many causes, including the normal aging process. Surgery, radiation to the pelvis, hormonal therapy, side effects from cancer treatments, or the cancer itself can all cause erectile dysfunction. Stress, fatigue, decreased sex drive, and body image issues may also contribute to erectile dysfunction.

Some cancer surgeries in the pelvis may require removing a nerve that is responsible for getting and maintaining an erection. There are now "nerve-sparing" surgeries that will increase your chance of getting and maintaining an erection.

You should speak to your doctor or nurse if you are having difficulty getting or maintaining an erection. They may perform a blood test to check your hormone levels. The course of treatment will depend on the results of a physical exam, blood tests, and your medical and sexual history. Prescription medications available to treat erectile dysfunction include Viagra®, Levitra®, and Cialis®. Vacuum constriction devices, penile injections, and penile implants are also possible options available to treat erectile dysfunction. Your doctor will help you decide on the best option for you.

76. Am I allowed to drink alcohol while receiving treatment?

This depends on your treatment regimen, your extent of disease, and your level of fatigue. Ask your doctor what he or she recommends in terms of your alcohol intake. Remember that alcohol in excess is dangerous to anyone, especially someone with a cancer diagnosis, so be sure to discuss alcohol intake with your doctor, as it may affect your blood test results, side effects, and treatment efficacy.

77. What causes fatigue with cancer treatments?

Fatigue may be caused by a number of factors, including the following:

- Chemotherapy medications
- Destruction of cancer cells
- Antinausea medications
- Infection
- Fever
- Pain
- Poor nutrition
- Injury to normal cells
- Anemia
- Shortness of breath

There are many techniques that may help manage fatigue.

- It is essential that you discuss your side effects with your health care providers so that they can take the appropriate steps to ensure that you can function at your optimum level while undergoing treatment.
- Plan a routine that enables you to do what you can when you feel energized, rest when necessary, and schedule your activities for the times when you are feeling energetic.

Remember that alcohol in excess is dangerous to anyone, especially someone with a cancer diagnosis, so be sure to discuss alcohol intake with your doctor, as it may affect your blood test results, side effects, and treatment efficacy.

• Discuss your needs with family and friends, and do not hesitate to ask for help from those closest to you.

Try to maintain a nutritious diet. This may be difficult, but it is essential to eat small, frequent meals that are protein-rich and well balanced. You may wish to seek the help of a nutritionist to help you achieve these goals.

78. How do I handle fatigue that comes with and after cancer treatment?

Fatigue is a common side effect for people undergoing cancer treatments, and it is experienced when you feel tired after exertion and, for many, even with minimal or no exertion. Fatigue can be severe and varies from person to person.

People receiving cancer treatments that include chemotherapy, radiation, surgery, or any combination of these therapies may complain of fatigue. Fatigue is a common side effect for people undergoing cancer treatments, and it is experienced when you feel tired after exertion and, for many, even with minimal or no exertion. Fatigue can be severe and varies from person to person. There is no true indicator for fatigue, and it can be gradual or sudden. Sleeping more at night, by going to bed earlier and waking up later, will help improve your energy. Resting during the day, napping, or just lying down and relaxing will all help your energy level. For some, simple tasks such as eating, bathing, and dressing can make you feel tired. Do not exhaust yourself, but keep in mind that inactivity may also lead to weakness. Exercise has been shown to increase your energy level. It is important to find a good balance by adjusting the intensity and frequency of your exercise workout based on the way you feel.

Ask your doctor about medications to help your fatigue. A common cause of fatigue in cancer patients is anemia (a drop in the red blood cells). There are very good drugs available to improve anemia, including Aranesp®, Epogen®, and oral and intravenous iron.

Sometimes it can be very difficult to treat fatigue. Often, the best way to manage it, therefore, is to simply adjust your activity level based upon what you feel you are able to do.

Ann's comment:

I was surprised at how long it took to feel wiped out from the treatment. The chemo alone wasn't bad at all; I only started to feel really tired a few weeks into the 5-week course of radiation and chemo. Most days, I tried to take a walk since I knew it would help fight fatigue. I didn't cook much, but there are lots of stores near our apartment that sell very good, healthy prepared food. I declined most, if not all, social invitations. I watched a lot of videos and DVDs. And I relied on our answering machine to field all the phone calls I didn't have the energy to answer. Eventually, either my husband or I returned the calls and let people know how I was doing.

79. What happens if I don't have any side effects? How do I know if my treatment is working?

It is possible to have treatments and have few side effects and in some cases have no side effects at all. It is important to know that side effects are cumulative, and what you do not experience in early treatments can occur later as you are exposed to more and more treatments. Be aware that at some point in your treatment cycle you will experience some side effects even if in their mildest form. The likelihood of eventual side effects is also dependent on the time frame of your treatments. For example, if you are undergoing 4 to 6 months of treatment, it is possible that you could have minimal side effects, while the patient undergoing life-long therapy could experience multiple side effects at various points in the treatment cycle. It is also important to know that the side effect guidelines for each specific treatment plan are just that—guidelines. Some patients will have all or most side effects, and some patients will have next to none. Side effects are treatment- and patient-specific.

The best way to analyze whether treatments are working is through diagnostic testing in the form of CT scans, PET

Some patients will have all or most side effects, and some patients will have next to none. Side effects are treatment- and patient-specific.

scans, and/or endoscopies. These diagnostic tests are ordered at specific intervals during the treatment cycles. These various tests tell specifically whether the cancer has increased in size, decreased in size, stayed the same, or spread to other parts of the body. Most gastric cancer patients have some sort of symptomology with their disease (for example, pain, inability to eat, difficulty swallowing, or recurrent vomiting); another subjective way to know that treatments are working is if the disease symptoms decrease or disappear with subsequent treatments.

80. Are there any alternative or complementary therapies that are recommended during treatment and recovery? Are vitamins or herbal supplements helpful?

Complementary and Alternative medicine (CAM) includes a wide array of treatments and approaches to treat disease and promote well-being that are not recognized as standard practices by the medical community. **Complementary medicine** is treatment used in addition to standard treatments. **Alternative therapy** is treatment used instead of standard treatment procedures. Acupuncture, massage therapy, herbal supplements, vitamins, and special diets are all types of complementary or alternative therapies. Many people believe that these alternative or complementary therapies make them feel better; however, some of them may actually change the way standard treatment works, and these changes could be harmful to your body. Many people with cancer try one or more kinds of alternative or complementary therapies, but usually without seeking the advice of their doctor. It is always best to consult your physician before you decide to try other therapies. Most of them are expensive and are generally not covered by insurance.

There are several reliable sources of information about complementary and alternative therapies.

Complementary medicine

Treatment used in addition to standard treatments.

Alternative medicine

Treatment used instead of standard treatment procedures.

- Memorial Sloan-Kettering Cancer Center at *www.mskcc.org/about herbs*.
- MD Anderson Cancer Center at *www.mdanderson.org/topics/complementary*.
- National Center for Complementary and Alternative Medicine of the National Institutes of Health at *nccam.nih.gov/health*.

There are many complementary methods that you can use safely along with standard treatments to help relieve symptoms or side effects of your disease and/or treatment. The following is a list of the most common:

- Acupuncture: Acupuncture is a technique in which very thin needles of varying lengths are inserted through the skin to treat a variety of conditions (such as pain and nausea).
- Aromatherapy: Aromatherapy is the use of fragrant substances, called essential oils, distilled from plants to alter mood or improve health.
- Art therapy: Art therapy is used to help people with physical and emotional problems by using creative activities to express emotions.
- Biofeedback: Biofeedback uses monitoring devices to help people consciously control physical processes such as heart rate, blood pressure, temperature, sweating, and muscle tension, all of which are usually controlled automatically.
- Massage therapy: Massage involves manipulation, rubbing, and kneading of the body's muscle and soft tissue. Some recent studies suggest massage can decrease stress, anxiety, depression, and pain, and can increase alertness.
- Meditation: Meditation is a mind-body process that uses concentration or reflection to relax the body and calm the mind.

- Music therapy: Music therapy is offered by established health care professionals who use music to promote healing and enhance quality of life.
- Prayer and spirituality: Spirituality is generally described as an awareness of something greater than the individual self. It is often expressed through religion and/or prayer, although there are many other paths of spiritual pursuit and expression.
- Tai chi: Tai chi is an ancient Chinese martial art. It is a mind-body, self-healing system that uses movement, meditation, and breathing to improve health and well-being.
- Yoga: Yoga is a form of nonaerobic exercise that involves a program of precise posture and breathing activities. In ancient Sanskrit, the word yoga means "union."

Ann's comment:

I've always been interested in alternative therapies like massage, acupuncture, and Chinese medicine, including nutritional approaches to disease. But I was wary of interfering with the medical treatment I was receiving; I didn't want to do anything that would jeopardize its effectiveness. Even though I really wanted to try drinking freshly squeezed vegetable juices—they were recommended by a cancer survivor I knew—I couldn't stand the taste. In the end, I just tried to eat healthy and nutritious foods. The only supplement I took other than my prescription medications was a multivitamin, and only after my oncologist said it was okay.

81. Will I be able to work during and after treatment?

If you feel excited and energized about your work or if you enjoy the camaraderie at work, you will probably want to continue working during your treatment. Some patients find that working allows them to retain some normalcy in their lives, in addition to allowing them to concentrate on something other than themselves, their disease, and their treatment. Many people feel well during their treatment and are able to continue working, either full-time or part-time.

However, some people do not feel well enough and must make adjustments in their hours or functions at work. Ask your physician how you should expect to feel during treatment and his or her recommendation regarding your working. Response to chemotherapy varies greatly from one person to another. Chemotherapy is usually given on an outpatient basis, either in one day or over several days each week. Some patients are able to work while receiving chemotherapy, while others find it necessary to take some time off from work.

Radiation therapy is given Monday through Friday. Treatment lasts for only a few minutes, but travel time to and from the hospital must be taken into account. Patients who have surgery usually require a 10- to 14-day hospital stay and a 6- to 8- week recovery period before they resume working. Discuss your treatment plan with your physician so that you can estimate how much time off you will need.

Discussing your diagnosis with your boss and coworkers can be an anxiety-provoking experience. People who continue to work are often unsure about whether to tell anyone about their cancer diagnosis, whom to tell, and how much to tell. Under the Americans with Disabilities Act, you are protected from discrimination at work. This act requires employers to make reasonable adjustments as long as you can perform the necessary tasks required of your job. If you need to speak to your supervisor or coworker, practice and prepare your conversation ahead of time. Being open and honest about your needs will be helpful in getting information about your rights and benefits. You will need to determine how you will perform the most important functions of your job. You will also have to devise a schedule so that you can balance your work hours

Ask your physician how you should expect to feel during treatment and his or her recommendation regarding your working. Response to chemotherapy varies greatly from one person to another.

Discussing your diagnosis with your boss and coworkers can be an anxiety-provoking experience. People who continue to work are often unsure about whether to tell anyone about their cancer diagnosis, whom to tell, and how much to tell.

with those that you will need for your medical care. If you are unable to speak to your supervisor or coworker, talk with someone in your company's human resources department. For more information on the Americans with Disabilities Act, contact the U.S. Department of Justice at 1-800-514-0301 or the U.S. Equal Employment Opportunity Commission at 1-202-663-4900.

It is possible to work during and after treatment if your side effects are minimal and your energy level is sufficient. Working is also a possibility if you are able to work out a flexible schedule that allows you time off for treatments and days when you may be too fatigued to go into the office. Anything that allows patients to feel good about themselves and is not detrimental to their health, well-being, or treatment is always encouraged.

Jim's comment:

I continued my normal daily routine as much as possible during my chemotherapy. My worst period was between the end of my chemo and radiation and before my surgery. I was told that there was a 4- to 6-week rest period between my treatments and my surgery. At first I did not understand the need for this rest period, but it became apparent when the accumulated effects began to manifest themselves. During the time between the radiation and the surgery, I was on four pain medications, and I got an infection at my port that resulted in a short hospital stay. When I look back, I certainly understand the need to regain your strength prior to the surgery. And, of course, there was the down time after my surgery. I tried to become active as fast as I could after the surgery, but everyone should take as long as it takes to recuperate from everything that is happening to your body. Even today, four years later, there are periods when I limit my activities, but this is a result of my anemia.

82. How do I manage the financial restraints that cancer places on our family?

When someone is diagnosed and treated for cancer, the financial burdens placed on the family can be overwhelming. Many patients appoint a family member or friend to be in charge of the financial issues that may arise. The first step is to review the patient's insurance benefits. If you are not clear about the benefits, speak to the insurance company directly to clear up any confusing issues. Questions that are important to ask include:

- What hospitals are covered under this plan?
- What doctors can treat this person? Does this person have to see a physician in the network? How much will you have to pay if you see an out-of-network physician?
- Does the plan pay for a second opinion?
- Do you need prior authorization for certain lab and diagnostic tests?
- What prescription medications are covered under this plan?
- Is home health care covered under this plan, and which agency do you have to use?

Be sure to meet with a financial counselor at the hospital to determine the estimated cost of care, and discuss a payment plan for those expenses that may be out of pocket. If you are unable to meet these financial obligations, meet with a social worker to find out what financial assistance may be available.

Many pharmaceutical companies provide assistance programs to give you medication at a reduced cost. Ask your nurse or social worker if the pharmaceutical company that makes the required medication has a financial assistance program.

Keep an accurate log of all financial costs incurred as a result of cancer and treatment. Speak to the accountant to find out which expenses are tax deductible and what receipts you should keep. Medical costs not covered by insurance (copays and deductibles), health insurance policy costs, and out-of-pocket expenses (transportation costs and medication costs) are tax deductible for most people.

Cancer treatment costs vary depending on the type of treatment, how long it lasts, how often it is given, and whether you are treated at home or treated in a clinic, office, or hospital. Most health plans cover at least part of the cost of many treatments. In many states, Medicaid may help pay for certain treatments. Before you begin treatment, find out whether your insurance company, Medicaid, or Medicare will pay for your care. Find out also what part of the expense, if any, will be your responsibility. Learning about your health insurance will help you prepare not only for the expense of treatment, but also for the process of talking or writing to the many people involved in helping to manage your health insurance plan. Patients who understand their insurance and know how to work with the insurance company are more likely to be successful in getting the coverage they need. Sometimes it is necessary to go outside the plan for the cancer care that is best for you.

Most health plans cover at least part of the cost of many treatments. In many states, Medicaid may help pay for certain treatments. Before you begin treatment, find out whether your insurance company, Medicaid, or Medicare will pay for your care.

83. How do I determine what information on the Internet is current and correct?

With the Internet, you can have instant access to an enormous amount of information without leaving your home. But because the information posted on the Internet is not regulated, you should be wary of its accuracy. Looking for specific topics on a Web site will help you determine whether the site's information is accurate and current. Always ascertain the sponsor of the site; consider whether the sponsor benefits by presenting a biased point of view. Other sites may be run by medical centers, hospitals, pharmaceutical companies, government agencies, or nonprofit organizations, so determine the purpose of the site—it should be clearly stated. Determine the source of information and whether the credentials are reliable. Review the credentials and affiliations to make sure they are truly experts in the field. Always look for information to back up any scientific research findings. Many Web sites may cite published articles as a source of information. Always check the date the information was reviewed and updated; this will ensure that you are getting current information. Before acting on any information you get from the Internet, always discuss your options with your physician.

84. When am I cured of stomach cancer?

For localized disease, the treatment may include surgery with or without chemotherapy, or chemotherapy with radiation (see Part 5, Treatment Options). Following surgery and any additional therapy, there is a chance that your cancer can return or recur. The chance is highest in the first 2 years following surgery and reduces with each consecutive year. After about 5 years post surgery, the chance for a recurrence is very, very small (less than 2% to 3%).

For cancer that has spread beyond the stomach, the primary treatment will be chemotherapy (as discussed in Part 5, Treatment Options). Unfortunately, for most patients with metastatic disease, the cancer will not go away completely. However, for some patients, particularly if the biology of their cancer is sensitive to chemotherapy treatment, there is a chance that the cancer can completely respond to treatment. In the rare event that the cancer is completely resolved with chemotherapy alone, the chance for recurrence also diminishes with time. Almost all of the time, the cancer will recur within 1 to 2 years following completion of the chemotherapy. Once again, after about 5 years post chemotherapy, the chance of recurrence of stomach cancer becomes very, very small (less than 2% to 3%).

85. How can I cope with the fear of recurrence?

Having feelings of fear or anxiety that your cancer may come back is normal, so you should try not to feel guilty or criticize yourself if you experience them. There are strategies to help you cope with these feelings.

Cancer recurrence is when your cancer has returned after treatment and a period of time when no cancer was detected. The same cancer may come back in the same place it first started or in another place in the body. Having feelings of fear or anxiety that your cancer may come back is normal, so you should try not to feel guilty or criticize yourself if you experience them. There are strategies to help you cope with these feelings. Talk to someone you trust. Joining a support group and talking to survivors who experience the same fears and anxieties as you is a good way to explore your thoughts and feelings. Discuss your fears with your physician. Being knowledgeable is a good way to relieve unnecessary fears. The same coping strategies that you used when you went through treatment may also help you now. If none of these strategies work, talk with your doctor about a referral to a social worker, psychologist, or psychiatrist. They will help you find ways to cope with this anxiety and stress. You should not let the fear of cancer recurrence control your life because you have no control over it. There are a few tools that many people have used to help control their fears of recurrence.

- Always be informed. Being aware of what you can do for your health allows you to maintain a sense of control.
- Allow yourself to feel scared and uncertain, and articulate these fears. For many people, if they are able to express such strong feelings, then they are able to let them go.
- Maintain a positive attitude. Focus on wellness and what you can do to stay as healthy as possible.
- Make healthy lifestyle choices (for example, stop smoking, start exercising, learn to relax).
- Get support from family, friends, and support groups as necessary.

Ann's comment:

For me, one of the hardest things about the cancer is the constant fear of a recurrence. Thirty months after being diagnosed, I began going to a support group for cancer survivors. It was illuminating because I realized that there are people who are just as fearful as I am. I've also seen a psychiatrist and a cognitive therapist, but not on a regular basis. My mother has been a great help to me because she is the most determinedly upbeat person I know. Both her parents died of cancer when she was 5, and she was successfully treated for lymphoma in her 50s. She's now almost 81, and she tells me, when I'm feeling down, that she just knows I'm going to make it—and of course, I believe her. The other person who's been a bulwark is my husband. When I start worrying, he tells me in the most matter-of-fact way that I simply couldn't be doing all the activities I'm doing if I were sick. I guess it's a combination of things that keeps the anxiety at bay: having loving and supportive family members and friends; staying busy with work, travel, exercise, and cooking; indulging in simple pleasures like watching TV and going shopping; and, when all else fails, taking anti-anxiety medication. I think the longer I'm free of cancer, the less I'll worry about a recurrence.

86. Will I be able to do the things that I love, such as traveling and playing sports?

You will be able to do as many of your favorite activities as you want, although you may need to modify them during treatment depending on how you feel. You should try to maintain your normal routine as closely as possible. A good cancer treatment program will add to the quantity of your life in addition to maintaining the quality of life you had prior to developing cancer.

Exercising is a great way of building and maintaining strength while receiving treatment. Start slowly and increase to your level of comfort. Exercise with a partner in case you need anything. As long as you are physically able and mentally willing, participate in light to moderate exercise, sports, and/or any other activity that is not physically or mentally detrimental to your health management—as the saying goes, just do it. As always, feel free to discuss your health concerns with your health care team.

Jim's comment:

I do everything I have always done, except I can no longer scuba dive. So snorkeling is what I can do. Concentrate on the positives—you are alive!

87. Will I be able to get life insurance after I've been diagnosed with cancer?

Policies for life insurance are based on age, occupation, and health status. Life insurance companies measure risk of death, so having a preexisting medical condition like cancer makes it unlikely that they will cover you for life. Many insurance companies will insure you if you have been healthy for at least 5 years following a cancer diagnosis.

Some insurance companies specialize in insuring individuals with preexisting medical conditions. They may want to know the specific type of cancer, treatment, dates of treatment, and whether the cancer has metastasized. They may require you to submit copies of your medical records for proof of your situation. You should look for a company that has an "A" or better rating by A.M. Best (*www.ambest.com*). You should always check with the insurance carrier because some cases can be evaluated on an individual basis. If you are still working or retired, check with your human resources department to find out whether they provide coverage as part of your normal benefits.

Buying life insurance after a cancer diagnosis is challenging, but it is not necessarily impossible. Insurance companies have differing procedures and philosophies on offering life insurance policies to cancer survivors. Coverage decisions depend greatly on the size, type, and location of your tumor. When a policy is issued, the first premiums will be high because that is the time of greatest risk to the insurance company. For most cancers, as time passes, the risk of the cancer returning is lower. Most insurers will not offer a policy to someone who is still undergoing treatment for cancer. If you have been cancer-free for a few years, there's a good chance you can buy life insurance, although you might have to pay higher premiums. These higher premiums will usually disappear after a given period of time. Some insurers prefer to account for the risk of cancer recurring by charging higher premiums for only a few years, while others will impose smaller premium increases over a longer period of time or until the applicant has remained cancer-free for at least 10 years.

88. What are advanced care directives?

Advanced care directives are legal documents with specific instructions, prepared in advance, that are intended to direct a person's medical care if he or she becomes unable to do so in the future. Advanced care directives can take many forms. Laws about advanced care directives are different in each state, so you should be aware of the laws in your state.

A good advanced care directive describes the kind of treatment you would want depending on how sick you are. For example, the directive would describe what kind of care you want if you have an illness from which you are unlikely to recover or if you are permanently unconscious. Advanced directives usually tell your doctor that you don't want certain kinds of treatment. However, they can also say that you want a certain treatment no matter how ill you are. Examples of advanced directives include living wills, Do Not Resuscitate orders, and health care proxy.

Advanced care directive

A legal document with specific instructions, prepared in advance, that are intended to direct a person's medical care if he or she becomes unable to do so in the future.

Living will

A written, legal document that describes the kind of medical or life-sustaining treatments you would want if you were seriously or terminally ill.

A **living will** is a written, legal document that describes the kind of medical or life-sustaining treatments you want if you are seriously or terminally ill. This document explains which medical interventions you want to have performed and which you want withheld depending on the circumstances. There are a number of medical interventions that you may want to specify in a living will, including whether you want to receive nutrition through a feeding tube, be resuscitated, or have your heart shocked.

A DNR is a written request placed in your medical chart that states you do not want cardiopulmonary resuscitation (CPR) if your heart stops or if you stop breathing. Unless a DNR order is written, it is standard protocol to resuscitate any patient whose heart has stopped or who has stopped breathing.

When you make these decisions, it is important to understand the problems that could occur. If a problem is reversible, you may want to use all medical measures to treat and sustain life. If you have a problem that can no longer be controlled (progressive cancer), you may not want to take measures to support your life. In this situation, you may request a Do Not Resuscitate (DNR) order. A DNR is a written request placed in your medical chart that states you do not want cardiopulmonary resuscitation (CPR) if your heart stops or if you stop breathing. Unless a DNR order is written, it is standard protocol to resuscitate any patient whose heart has stopped or who has stopped breathing. You can use an advanced directive form or tell your doctor that you don't want to be resuscitated.

There are some limitations to a living will. A living will does not let you select someone to make decisions for you, and not all states recognize a living will. It is also very difficult to anticipate all the circumstances that may occur regarding your health. It is likely that problems will arise that have not been specified in writing. To avoid this problem, one can designate a health care proxy.

Health care proxy

A person who will make health care decisions for you if you are unable to do so.

A **health care proxy** (medical proxy, medical power of attorney, health care surrogate) designates a person who will make health care decisions for you if you are unable to. This person decides which treatments should be given or withheld. When choosing a health care proxy, choose someone whom you trust that will make decisions based on what you would want for yourself. This would be someone who knows you well, such as a friend or family member. You should talk to that person to make sure he or she understands what you would want in many different circumstances. Be sure to let your family and friends know whom you've chosen as your health care proxy. Keep in mind that you can change your designated health care proxy at any point during your treatment. All states recognize a health care proxy.

89. How can I talk to my friends and family about my diagnosis of cancer?

Having cancer can cause feelings of loneliness and alienation, or feelings that it is time to surround yourself with close friends and family. Talking to your friends and family openly about your cancer can make an enormous difference in how you handle this difficult time in your life. It will allow others to provide you support and help you overcome your feelings of loneliness. You can decide what thoughts and feelings you would like to share, and which ones you would like to keep private.

Some friends and family members may be afraid, uneasy, or apprehensive in hearing about your diagnosis. They may alienate themselves from you because of their own fears about cancer or because they are unsure of what to say to you. If this occurs, you may want to tell them that you miss them or would like to see them more often. You may find that some people will disappoint you, while others will surprise you in their willingness to help and support you.

If you are feeling pressured by your family and friends to talk about your diagnosis before you are ready, tell them that you just need a little time and that you appreciate their concern. Instead of pushing them away, reassure them that you will speak to them when you are ready. Most people find it helpful to be direct and honest when telling people about their cancer.

Some friends and family members may be afraid, uneasy, or apprehensive in hearing about your diagnosis. They may alienate themselves from you because of their own fears about cancer or because they are unsure of what to say to you.

If you have children, you may feel that you want to protect them from the news that you have cancer. It is much better that they hear it from you than overhear it from someone else. Children cope better when they are informed. Be open and honest when you speak to them. Select words that are age appropriate, and practice what you want to say before you sit down with them. Break down the information for them and encourage them to ask questions. Describe your disease and treatment and let them know how it will affect them. Talk about how their routine and activities may be affected.

There are many resources available to help children cope with cancer. KidsCope, at *www.kidscope.org*, is a Web site that helps children deal with the effects of cancer. The American Cancer Society has published several books on this topic, including *Our Mom Has Cancer* and *Cancer in the Family: Helping Children Cope with a Parent's Illness*.

People diagnosed with cancer may wonder who to tell and how to tell them. They often feel pressured to share their diagnosis, but most people are able to wait until they are ready.

People diagnosed with cancer may wonder who to tell and how to tell them. They often feel pressured to share their diagnosis, but most people are able to wait until they are ready. Many cannot anticipate how long it will be before they feel comfortable enough to discuss their cancer with others. There are no absolute rights and wrongs when dealing with people, because everyone copes differently. However, there a few tips (American Cancer Society) that can help you when telling family and friends about your diagnosis:

- Tell your friends and family what is going on. They will learn, sooner or later, that you have cancer.
- If you or your family members usually don't like to talk about certain personal issues, it's okay not to open up completely to everyone.
- Explain what kind of cancer you have, which treatments will be necessary, and that a cancer diagnosis is not a death sentence.
- Explain that cancer is not contagious (they can't catch it).

- Find out what they feel, and try to answer their questions.
- It is usually easier to express emotions than to hide them. Having other people know will help you and your and loved ones share strength and concern, to your mutual benefit.
- It is okay to wonder, "Why me?" or to feel sad. These feelings are normal and change as time goes on.
- Tell people that you'd rather not talk at a particular time if you don't feel up to it just then. Sometimes family members can do that for you.
- Realize that you may be a target for anger, but that you are not the cause. Anger is sometimes the first way people express fear.
- It is okay to be direct with others and to express your needs and feelings.
- Your role in your family will probably need to change so you can focus on treatment. You may not be able to do all that you have been doing.
- Allow friends and family to help you, but be specific about the kind of help you need.
- As much as possible, try to keep a sense of normalcy in your family while you are receiving treatment. Your family should try to keep doing the things they always did (playing bridge, fishing, exercising, playing basketball) without a sense of guilt.
- Get help if you feel overwhelmed. Ask your nurse, doctor, or minister for help or for a referral. You can also contact your local unit of the American Cancer Society.
- Many patients and their families find it very helpful to attend support groups for individuals facing cancer.

Jim's comment:

The second paragraph is so true. This was the area of my greatest surprise. Some people immediately write you off and others have no idea how to talk to you. It is almost like you become "contagious." There are so many people who do not know anything other than cancer is a killer. My advice is to open up the subject yourself, because most people don't know how or what to say; therefore, they are uncomfortable about bringing the subject up in conversation. You will have to gauge how much is the right amount to share with them. Some want to know everything, while others don't want many details. My wife had an e-mail list that she e-mailed regularly about my progress, and it really helped everyone. She and I didn't have to tell the same story over and over, and everyone didn't have to call constantly to get an update.

90. Should I be worried about becoming addicted to pain medication?

Studies show that it is rare for patients with cancer to develop addiction from taking pain medications. Taking pain medication does not cause addiction, but when taken on a regular basis, it does cause tolerance. Tolerance is when your body adjusts to the level of medication in your blood. This means that after a certain point, a greater amount of medication is needed to produce the same effect in the body. If you stop taking a medication suddenly, you may develop withdrawal symptoms. Reducing or tapering down your dose of medication slowly, rather than stopping it, can prevent this. Your doctor or nurse will discuss an appropriate regimen for you.

Addiction

A desire or craving for a substance to feel high.

Drug addiction

A dependence on the regular use of opioid analgesics to satisfy physical, emotional, and psychological needs rather than for medical reasons.

Tolerance to medication is not addiction. **Addiction** is a desire or craving for a substance to feel high. Fear of addiction is very common for people who take narcotics or opioid analgesics for pain relief. **Drug addiction** is defined as dependence on the regular use of opioid analgesics to satisfy physical, emotional, and psychological needs rather than for medical reasons. Pain relief is a medical reason for taking narcotics. Therefore, if you take opioid analgesics to relieve pain, you are not an "addict," regardless of how much or how often you take medicines. Drug addiction in cancer patients is rare and almost never occurs in people who do not have a history of drug abuse prior to illness.

PART SEVEN

Caring for Someone with Cancer

How can I cope with the burden of caring for my loved one?

What is the right thing to say to my loved one?

As a caregiver, how can I tell what is normal and what is urgent? When should I call the doctor for help?

More . . .

91. How can I cope with the burden of caring for my loved one?

When a person is diagnosed with cancer, tremendous demands are placed on family and friends. The stress will depend on the nature of the person who is ill: age, stage of the disease, type of treatment, symptoms, and the role that person plays in the family.

One demand placed on the caregiver is the need to provide physical care for the person who is ill. In recent years and with the advent of home health care, people can be cared for at home. This places the responsibility of care on family and friends. The demands may include ensuring the person is comfortable, administering medications, managing supplies and equipment, checking for signs and symptoms, and knowing when to call the doctor. As a person gets sicker, he or she may need help with bathing, dressing, feeding, and walking.

Nonmedical aspects of care may also need to be addressed by the caregiver. This may include running errands, providing transportation, coordinating and scheduling appointments, and handling financial obligations. The caregiver may also have to take on the tasks that the person who is ill previously performed.

The stress and demands placed on caregivers may make them feel over-whelmed and feel a variety of emotions including anger, guilt, fear, and sadness. If you are a caregiver, it is important to find a way to care for yourself and attend to your emotional needs while taking care of the person who is ill.

The stress and demands placed on caregivers may make them feel overwhelmed and feel a variety of emotions including anger, guilt, fear, and sadness. If you are a caregiver, it is important to find a way to care for yourself and attend to your emotional needs while taking care of the person who is ill.

Donna's comment:

Some may think of it as a burden, but I never did. My husband used to tell people he did not have cancer, we had cancer. And that really pretty much sums it up. God gives us all incredible strength when we need it and common sense to deal with the everyday challenges. The one thing I will say is that most people do not think of the stress that it does put on the caregiver or the loved ones. And trust me, there is stress. Sometimes the caregiver is not even aware of the stress, but there will be times that everyone needs some emotional support. Remember that friends and family offer to help because they want to do "something." Allow them to help in ways that also help you as the primary caregiver.

92. What is the right thing to say to my loved one who has cancer?

There is no correct answer to this question because no one answer works for everyone. It is difficult to know how best to help someone you love who has been diagnosed with cancer. You should try to anticipate what needs the person may have, and make specific offers to help support that need. Plan to be available on days when your loved one needs more help than usual; days when this person is ill or tired are especially good days to offer help. The things that you can offer to do are limitless, but a few examples include the following:

- Taking your loved one to a doctor's appointment or treatment center
- Dropping off a cooked meal
- Shopping for food and household items
- Helping with family obligations
- Cleaning the house and laundering the clothes

It is normal to feel unsure of the right things to say when someone you care about is diagnosed with cancer. You may feel nervous about asking simple questions about how he or she is doing because you are afraid you will not know how to respond to the answer. You may feel concerned about saying something hurtful, while unintentional. You may be worried that if you show your own sadness, this will cause the person to be upset. In dealing with your own discomfort, you may withdraw from the situation, distance yourself from the person, and call less often. But it is best not to do this, because

It is normal to feel unsure of the right things to say when someone you care about is diagnosed with cancer.

your avoidance will only leave the person feeling abandoned at a time when friends and family are needed the most.

The best way of helping is to offer your presence. You should match what you are able to do with the specific things that the person enjoys. It is important to consider their feelings and energy, and to not create unrealistic expectations for them. Make the time that you spend together pleasurable regardless of how long it is.

There are no guidelines to follow to help you know what to say. If you make assumptions about what the person is thinking or feeling, you may say things that will cause distress. The best way to start a conversation is by listening. Let the person know that you are there to listen if he or she would like to talk. Not everyone will want to share all of their feelings with those that they are close to. The important thing is to let the person know you are there to discuss as little or as much as he or she is willing to talk about.

It may be uncomfortable to hear about things that are distressing to those you love. You may feel like you want to change the subject or offer reassurance that things will be okay, even though this may not be true. This may help you deal with your own discomfort, but it generally doesn't help the person who wants to open up and share personal feelings. It is okay to simply tell your loved one that you are unsure of what to say and how to make him or her feel better.

Donna's comment:

Hearing the news that your loved one has cancer is always a blow to anyone. The dreaded "C" is something no one wants to hear. I am a strong believer in a positive attitude. From the moment my husband was diagnosed, I thought, "Okay, we have a big fight on our hands, and if that is what it takes, that is what we will do." I told my husband and the oncologist that even if the odds of survival are only 15%, that is not a problem, because we will be in the 15%. There are also a number of great books on the market written by cancer survivors, and I think they are definitely a comfort to the patient.

93. As a caregiver, how can I tell what is normal and what is urgent? When should I call the doctor for help?

As a caregiver, it is important that you ask the health care team what signs and symptoms should be reported. The caregiver's responsibility is to discuss all possible problems concerning treatment to the health care team, including any side effects that the patient may experience. In the event that you are unsure whether a particular symptom warrants a phone call to the doctor, it is always better to err on the side of caution and make the call. Always go with your gut feeling and address your concerns immediately to the members of the health care team. There is no such thing as a stupid question when one's health is involved.

Donna's comment:

I found that all medical staff were there for us when we needed answers. My only regret on some things was not asking a question sooner. Every patient reacts differently to his or her chemotherapy and radiation. Our bodies are wonderful alarm clocks, and they let us know when something is wrong—we just have to pay attention. No question is stupid, and no question is forbidden. Ask away. The more educated you are, the better; and remember that as the caregiver, you will remember far more than your patient will. I always took a pad and pen with me on each of our visits so I could ask the questions I had been thinking about, and so I could write down anything new the doctors had to share with us.

The caregiver's responsibility is to discuss all possible problems concerning treatment to the health care team, including any side effects that the patient may experience. In the event that you are unsure whether a particular symptom warrants a phone call to the doctor, it is always better to err on the side of caution and make the call.

PART EIGHT

Advocacy and Support

How do I prepare for worsening disease?

Are there support groups available?

What if my doctors suggest stopping my current treatment? What is the best supportive care?

More . . .

94. How do I prepare for worsening disease?

You can prepare for the prospect of your disease worsening by doing any of the following:

- Always stay educated about the nature of your illness.
- Always ask your health care team pertinent questions about your care.
- Prepare your affairs and finances while you are still healthy.
- Seek out psychosocial support from counselors and support groups to help cope with the issues of death and dying.
- Always ask your health care team about what to expect (that is, about the natural progression of disease) as you go through the stages of your cancer and treatment.
- Allow yourself to be sad.
- Try to maintain some normalcy in your life; visit the people you need to visit and make the trips that you have always wanted to make. Do not put things off until the last moment. Do as much as you want while you are mentally and physically able.
- Make peace with your life and your disease so that you may be able to enjoy the time that you have left.
- Keep positive and loving people in your circle so that you can maintain as positive an outlook as possible in the days that your disease begins to worsen.
- If you are a spiritual person, embrace your faith.

95. How do I prepare my family for my worsening disease?

If your disease is getting worse, you can prepare your family for what's ahead by doing the following:

- Do not keep your disease or extent of disease a secret from the people closest to you.

- Choose a family member to accompany you to your doctor visits so that this person is there with you to help you absorb the news of worsening disease.
- Sit down with family and/or friends who are closest to you and explain the extent of your disease and what you know to be the natural progression of it. By doing this, they are prepared and know what to expect as your condition worsens.
- Have those closest to you seek counseling services to help them cope with their emotions regarding your disease.
- Make peace with the people in your life who are most important.
- Spend quality time with your special loved ones.
- Do things with your family and friends closest to you. Make special memories so that after you are gone they will have these moments to remember and treasure.
- If there are young children in your life, make memory books with pictures, stories, and quotations that were important to you so that they can have these after you have passed on.
- Make video messages when you are feeling strong enough so that your loved ones can have them to look at after you have passed on.

96. Are there any support groups available?

Support groups give you the opportunity to share your thoughts and feelings with other patients with cancer. You can hear how other people have reacted and dealt with the same issues you may be facing. Support groups allow you to overcome feelings of alienation, or that no one really understands what you are going through.

Support groups are usually led by a trained patient leader or health professional. The group may be divided into specific types of cancer or be open to all who have cancer. Groups can

Support group

A gathering of people allowing you the opportunity to share your thoughts and feelings with other patients with cancer.

range from structured to very informal and relaxed. Some groups will also provide patient education by inviting speakers to talk about different topics. Groups may also decide on how to limit their members. They may only allow cancer patients to join or may allow families to participate as well. Selecting a support group that will be helpful to you is important.

A number of online support groups are available via the Internet, but remember that online support groups generally do not have professional involvement. Thus, the advice or information that you receive online may not always be accurate.

A number of online support groups are available via the Internet, but remember that online support groups generally do not have professional involvement. Thus, the advice or information that you receive online may not always be accurate. You should discuss any advice or information that you receive from these support groups with your doctor. Some online support is available at OncoChat *www.oncochat.org* and at Cancer Hope Network at *www.cancerhopenetwork.org*.

Donna's comment:

There are many, many advocacy and support groups available. Each one is a little different, and each one may have a different focus, but it shouldn't be hard for you to find one or more than one that fits your needs. You should be able to speak directly with a survivor and a caregiver, male or female, and no questions are off limits.

97. Are there any support groups available to help my significant other, family, and friends cope?

Just as the cancer patient may benefit from support groups, family members may also benefit from them. It may be beneficial to talk to other families who are going through similar experiences. Talking to a trained professional may also be useful. Some support groups are specifically for family and friends of people diagnosed with cancer. Other support groups encourage patients and family members to take part in the same group. The National Cancer Institute (NCI) provides information for people with cancer that lists organizations that provide support groups. This is available online at *cis.nci.nih.gov/fact/8_1.htm*, or you can call the Cancer Information Service at 1-800-4-CANCER.

Donna's comment:

Yes, many advocacy groups have support for loved ones and caregivers.

98. What if my doctors suggest stopping my current therapy? What is best supportive care?

If your cancer becomes too advanced and resistant to therapy, or if your body becomes too weak to tolerate treatment, your doctor may decide to stop all active therapies. You may feel angry, upset, or helpless as a result. This does not mean that your doctor is giving up on your treatment; rather, he or she is trying to protect you from any further harm from treatment that may no longer be beneficial against your cancer. Your doctor will concentrate on the best supportive care available. **Best supportive care** is therapy geared toward alleviating symptoms, and it is still considered an active treatment approach. You will still see your doctor regularly. You will discuss pain management, nutrition, abdominal discomfort, and other symptoms or concerns that you may have. Controlling these symptoms will allow you to maintain some functional existence at this stage of your disease. You should use this time to spend with your family and friends, enjoy hobbies, visit places you enjoy, or attend religious services. Keeping a positive attitude is the key to success in this unusually difficult time.

Best supportive care

Therapy geared toward alleviating symptoms; it is still considered an active treatment approach.

99. What is hospice care?

Hospice care recognizes death as the final stage of life and seeks to enable patients to continue an alert, pain-free life. Hospice care addresses medical, physical, social, emotional, and spiritual needs for patients with advanced disease. Hospice allows for those last days to be spent with dignity and quality, surrounded by family and loved ones. Hospice focuses on controlling the pain and suffering of a patient with a cancer diagnosis when active and aggressive cancer treatment is no

Hospice care

Care designed to give supportive care to people in the final phase of a terminal illness.

longer an option. Hospice affirms life and neither hastens nor postpones death. Hospice care treats the person rather than the disease; it emphasizes quality of life rather than quantity of life. It provides family-centered care that involves both the patient and family in making decisions. Although the hospice team may be present at your home for only a few hours a day, care is provided for the patient and family 24 hours a day, 7 days a week. Hospice care can be given in the patient's home, a hospital, a nursing home, or a private hospice facility. If possible, it is preferable to provide hospice care in the home, with family members serving as the main hands-on caregivers.

Hospice care is appropriate when you can no longer benefit from aggressive cancer treatment and life expectancy is, at most, no longer than 6 months. You, your family, and your doctor decide together when hospice services should begin.

Hospice care is appropriate when you can no longer benefit from aggressive cancer treatment and life expectancy is, at most, no longer than 6 months. You, your family, and your doctor decide together when hospice services should begin. If your condition improves or the disease goes into remission, you can be discharged from the hospice program and return to active cancer treatment, if desired.

Whether hospice care is managed at home or in a hospital, nursing home, or private hospice facility, the care is managed by a health care team that comprises physicians, nurses, caregivers, social workers, and sometimes trained volunteers who manage the patient's pain and symptoms. They also assist with the emotional, psychosocial, and spiritual needs of the patient and family as they go through the dying process. Hospice services include providing medications and the necessary supplies for care. The hospice team also teaches the family how to care for the patient while providing bereavement counseling to the family and loved ones of the deceased.

100. Where can I go to find more information?

The information in this book cannot answer all of the questions you might have. The accompanying appendix offers a selection of good resources to address many topics and resources. As always you should use your health professional team as a resource too.

Appendix

Organizations

American Cancer Society

www.cancer.org

phone 1-800-ACS-2345

The American Cancer Society (ACS) is a nationwide, community-based voluntary health organization. Headquartered in Atlanta, Georgia, the ACS has state divisions and more than 3,400 local offices. Their mission statement is as follows:

> *The American Cancer Society is the nationwide community-based voluntary health organization dedicated to eliminating cancer as a major health problem by preventing cancer, saving lives, and diminishing suffering from cancer, through research, education, advocacy, and service.*

American Society of Clinical Oncology

www.asco.org

phone 703-299-0150

E-mail: asco@asco.org

The American Society of Clinical Oncology is the world's largest cancer organization for physicians who treat cancer patients. Although ASCO supports all types of cancer research, its primary interest is in patient-oriented clinical research.

National Cancer Institute

www.cancer.gov

phone 1-800-4-CANCER

This Web site offers accurate, up-to-date, comprehensive cancer information from the U.S. government's principal agency for cancer research.

Hereditary Diffuse Gastric Cancer

HDGC@yahoogroups.com

This is a group for families with Hereditary Diffuse Gastric Cancer, their caregivers, and medical professionals working to understand, prevent, and treat the disease.

Selected Cancer Center Web Sites

Mayo Clinic
www.MayoClinic.com

MD Anderson Cancer Center
www.mdanderson.org

Memorial Sloan-Kettering Cancer Center
www.mskcc.org

Dana-Farber Cancer Institute
www.dana-farber.org

Survivorship and Family Resources

National Coalition for Cancer Survivorship
www.canceradvocacy.org
The National Coalition for Cancer Survivorship is the oldest survivor-led cancer advocacy organization in the country and a highly respected authentic voice at the federal level, advocating for quality cancer care for all Americans and empowering cancer survivors.

Corporate Angel Network
www.corpangelnetwork.org
phone 914-328-1313
fax 914-328-3938
toll-free patient line is 866-328-1313
The Corporate Angel Network arranges free air transportation for cancer patients traveling to treatment by using empty seats on corporate jets.

National Alliance for Caregiving
www.caregiving.org
4720 Montgomery Lane, 5th floor, Bethesda, MD 20814
The National Alliance for Caregiving is a national nonprofit organization dedicated to providing support to family caregivers and the professionals who help them, and to increasing public awareness of issues facing family caregivers.

National Family Caregivers Association

www.nfcacares.org

phone 1-800-896-3650 or 301-942-6430

fax 301-942-2302

The National Family Caregivers Association educates, supports, empowers, and speaks up for the more than 50 million Americans who care for loved ones with a chronic illness or disability or the frailties of old age. NFCA reaches across the boundaries of diagnoses, relationships, and life stages to address the common needs and concerns of all family caregivers.

Cancer Care

www.cancercare.org

phone 1-800-813-HOPE

Cancer Care is a national nonprofit organization that provides free professional support services for anyone affected by cancer.

GastroEsophageal Cancer Foundation

www.gecancer.org

phone 281-320-0022

A not-for-profit organization that provides free support and counseling information to anyone affected by gastroesophageal cancer.

Glossary

A

Addiction: A desire or craving for a substance to feel high.

Adenocarcinoma: A type of cancer that begins from gland-forming or secretory cells.

Adjuvant chemoradiation: Chemotherapy and radiation given following curative intent surgery for locally advanced gastric or GEJ carcinomas.

Adjuvant therapy: Therapy to treat cancer that is given after surgery.

Advanced care directive: A legal document with specific instructions, prepared in advance, that are intended to direct a person's medical care if he or she becomes unable to do so in the future.

Alopecia: Hair loss.

Alternative medicine: Treatment used instead of standard treatment procedures.

Analgesics: Medications that treat pain.

Anthracyclines: An older class of chemotherapy drugs derived from antibiotics.

Anti-angiogenesis agents: Drugs that attack the blood vessels to tumors.

Antimetabolites: A class of chemotherapy that inhibits DNA synthesis, often by inhibiting the enzyme thymidylate synthase.

Antrum: The last portion of the stomach where food is mixed with gastric juices.

Apoptosis: Programmed cell death; the natural process by which cells kill themselves.

Ascites: An abnormal accumulation of fluid in the abdomen.

B

Benign tumor: A growth or mass of abnormal cells that do not invade or destroy adjacent normal tissue.

Best supportive care: Therapy geared toward alleviating symptoms; it is still considered an active treatment approach.

Biologic therapy: A treatment that uses the patient's immune system to fight cancer.

C

Cancer: An abnormal growth of cells which tends to proliferate in an uncontrolled way. It is a group of diseases that affect the normal cells of our body.

Cancer staging: The process to identify the extent of the cancer in the body. The stage is usually determined by the depth of penetration into the wall, the involvement of lymph nodes next to the cancer, and whether the cancer has traveled from the primary origin to metastatic sites of disease.

Carcinoid tumors: Tumors of hormone-producing cells of the stomach.

Cardia: The first portion of the stomach which overlaps with the junction between the stomach and esophagus.

Cell: The smallest unit of living structure capable of independent existence. Cells are highly specialized in structure and function.

Chemoradiation: Treatment that combines chemotherapy with radiation therapy.

Chemotherapy: A type of treatment for cancer that uses drugs to stop the growth of cancer cells, either by killing the cells or by stopping them from dividing.

Clinical trial: A research study that is designed to test a specific treatment on humans. This treatment may be a new drug, a new combination of drugs, radiation therapy, biologics, or a new drug for a different disease.

Complementary medicine: Treatment used in addition to standard treatments.

D

Depression: A medical condition in which the person suffering feels an intractable sense of loss or helplessness. Situational depression occurs as a result or consequence of a particular event or circumstance that occured.

Designer drugs: Drugs developed specifically to attack the cancer at a very specific and critical target or pathway.

Differentiation: When describing cancer, refers to how mature a cell appears under the microscope. The more differentiated the cancer cell, the more normal in appearance it is, and the slower it tends to grow. Poorly differentiated or undifferentiated cancer cells lack the structure and function of normal cells.

Diffuse Hereditary Gastric Cancer: A hereditary syndrome in which affected individuals have an increased risk of developing diffuse gastric cancer.

DNA: Deoxyribonucleic acid. A type of nucleic acid found principally in the nuclei of animal and plant cells; considered to be the autoreproducing component of chromosomes and many viruses as well as the repository for hereditary characteristics.

Drug addiction: A dependence on the regular use of opioid analgesics to satisfy physical, emotional, and psychological needs rather than for medical reasons.

Dumping syndrome: A group of symptoms that occur when food or liquid enters the small intestine too rapidly. These symptoms include cramps, nausea, diarrhea, and dizziness.

E

Endoluminal stent placement: A procedure to insert a stent (a thin, expandable tube) in order to keep a passage (such as arteries or the esophagus) open.

Endoscopic laser surgery: A procedure in which an endoscope (a thin, lighted tube) with a laser attached is inserted into the body.

Epidermal Growth Factor Receptor Inhibitors: A class of biologic drugs that block the signaling from a cellular receptor called the epidermal growth factor receptor.

Erectile dysfunction: The inability to have and/or maintain an erection.

Esophagus: A portion of the digestive canal, shaped like a hollow tube, that connects the throat to the stomach. It is a muscular tube that transfers the bolus of food from the mouth to the stomach. The bolus moves to the stomach independent of gravity—e.g., even if you stand on your head, the food you eat will end up in the stomach.

Esophagogastroduodenoscopy: An examination of the lining of the esophagus, stomach, and upper duodenum with a flexible tube that has a small camera on the end and that is inserted down the throat.

External radiation therapy: Radiation treatment that uses an external radiation source that is then directed or aimed at a specific position within the body.

F

Familial adenomatous polyposis (FAP): A hereditary syndrome that significantly increases the risk of colon cancer and also stomach cancer. It is characterized by thousands of polyps in the intestines.

5-year survival rate: The percentage of patients who live for at least 5 years after they are diagnosed with cancer.

Fundus: The second portion of the stomach which forms the bulk of the stomach.

G

Gastric lymphoma: Cancer of the immune system cells found in the stomach.

Gastroesophageal junction (GEJ): Where the esophagus and stomach meet. It contains the lower esophageal sphincter, which opens and closes, to prevent acid from refluxing into the esophagus.

Gastrointestinal stromal tumor (GIST): A type of tumor that begins from the cells within the wall of the gastrointestinal tract. Most tumors arise from within the wall of the stomach but can arise anywhere throughout the gastrointestinal tract.

H

Health care proxy: A person who will make health care decisions for you if you are unable to do so.

Heavy Metals: Metal based anticancer drugs that kill by causing crosslinks in DNA strands.

Helicobacter pylori (H. pylori): A bacteria that causes inflammation and irritation of the lining of the stomach and intestine. Infection with *H. pylori* can cause ulceration of the stomach and different types of stomach cancer, including gastric adenocarcinoma and MALT lymphoma.

Hereditary nonpolyposis colorectal cancer: A hereditary syndrome that significantly increases the risk of many cancers including the colon and stomach. Unlike FAP, it is not characterized by numerous polyps.

Home care: Health care provided in the patient's home by either health care professionals or by family and friends.

Home health care: Care provided by licensed and trained medical personnel.

Hospice care: Care designed to give supportive care to people in the final phase of a terminal illness.

I

Immune system: A collection of mechanisms that protects against infection by identifying and killing pathogens.

Interdisciplinary care: Range of disciplines (doctors, nurses, social workers, pharmacists, etc.) work together as a team at one facility to provide your health care.

Internal radiation therapy: Radiation treatment that uses a source that can be directly injected or inserted into a specific position within the body.

Intrinsic factor: Protein made by the parietal cells of the stomach to help the absorption of vitamin B_{12}. Its deficiency is associated with the development of pernicious anemia.

J

Jaundice: Yellowish discoloration of the skin and eyes caused by accumulation of bilirubin.

L

Laparoscopy: Examination of the interior of the abdomen by means of a laparoscope.

Living will: Written, legal document that describes the kind of medical treatments or life-sustaining treatments you would want if you were seriously or terminally ill.

Lymph nodes: Small, beanlike structures located all over the body that filter unwanted substances like bacteria from lymph.

M

Malignant tumor: A growth of abnormal cells that replace normal cells and invade other tissues and organs; growth may recur after attempted removal, and is likely to cause the death of the host if left inadequately treated.

Mediports/portocaths: Devices that access a central vein used for giving chemotherapy.

Menetrier disease: Hyperproliferative disorders of the stomach caused by dysregulated receptor tyrosine kinases (RTKs).

Metastasis: A term that describes the spread of cancer from one part of the body to another. A tumor formed by cells that have spread is called a "metastatic tumor" or a "metastasis." The tumor cells at a metastatic site contain cells that are like those of the primary cancer.

Mucosa: The inner layer of the stomach where the juices made by the glands help digest food.

Mucosa-Associated Lymphoid Tissue (MALT) Lymphoma: A type of cancer that originates from the lymph cells within the lining of the gastrointestinal tract responsible for making antibodies to pathogens. Most MALT lymphomas arise from the stomach and are often caused by infection with *H. pylori*.

Mucositis: Mouth sores that may occur with certain chemotherapy treatments.

Muscle layer: Creates the motion that is responsible for mixing and mashing food.

Myelosuppression: A condition in which bone marrow activity is decreased, resulting in fewer red blood cells, white blood cells, and platelets. Myelosuppression is a side effect of some cancer treatments.

N

Neoadjuvant therapy: Therapy to treat cancer that is given before surgery.

P

Palliative care: Care that is not curative and encompasses medical, physical, emotional, spiritual, and social well-being and is directed at helping patients achieve the best quality of life.

PCA pump: Patient controlled analgesic pump, whereby the patient determines when he or she needs some extra pain relief.

Peritoneum: The tissue that lines the abdominal wall and most of the structures and organs within the abdomen.

Photodynamic therapy: High intensity light treatment using a chemical photosensitizer to make the cancer cells sensitive to the treatment.

Polyps: A growth in the lining of the intestines. They come in a variety of shapes and carry a varying risk of developing into a cancer.

Primary cancer: Describes the site of origin of the cancer and generally is described by the organ in which it started.

R

Radiation therapy: A type of cancer treatment that uses high-energy x-rays or other types of radiation to kill cancer cells or keep them from growing.

Regional chemotherapy: Chemotherapy that is placed directly into the spinal column, organ, or body cavity to affect cells in a certain region or area.

Risk factor: Anything that increases a person's risk of getting a disease.

S

Second opinion: An extensive exam designed to get input and an opinion from a second physician.

Sporadic mutation: A genetic mutation that occurs the first time in the family or a new mutation that is not likely to occur again within the family.

Stem cells: Special cells that can turn into any other type of cell in the body.

Stomach: An organ of digestion. The stomach begins the digestion process by mixing food with digestive juices, churning it into a liquid mulch.

Stomach cancer/gastric cancer: The transformation of normal cells of the stomach into cancerous cells.

Submucosa: The support tissue for the inner layer of the stomach.

Subserosa: The support tissue for the outer layer of the stomach.

Support group: A gathering of people allowing you the opportunity to share your thoughts and feelings with other patients with cancer.

Systemic chemotherapy: Chemotherapy that is injected into a muscle or vein and subsequently enters the bloodstream. The chemotherapy reaches cancer cells via blood circulation.

T

Taxanes: A new class of anticancer drug that attacks microtubules.

Topoisomerase Inhibitors: A new class of chemotherapy that kills cancer cells by inhibiting an enzyme, topoisomerase I, involved in DNA repair.

Tumor: Any swelling caused by an increased number of abnormal cells.

U

Upper endoscopy: Examination of the inside of the stomach using an endoscope; a thin, tube-like instrument with a light and a lens for viewing; passed through the mouth and esophagus.

V

Vitamin B$_{12}$: An essential vitamin important in making red blood cells and DNA; helps with the normal functioning of the nervous system. Also known as cobalamin. Deficiency of vitamin B$_{12}$ can result in anemia, peripheral neuropathy with numbness and tingling in the fingertips and toes, loss of appetite, weight loss, and a sore tongue that can sometimes appear smooth and beefy red.

Index